The Diet Fallacies

Change Your Diet, Change Your Weight, End Food Cravings, and Transform Your Life!

Never Diet Again!

Al Davis

ISBN: 978-0-9978880-1-0

Disclaimer

Please note that I am not a doctor, nutritionist, or other health care professional, that the ideas in this book are opinions only, and are not to be considered or construed as medical advice.

It is <u>imperative</u> that you consult with your physician before beginning to eat in the way recommended in this book. If you take insulin, blood pressure medication, and blood thinners, following the plan will change your needs for these particular medications, and possibly others as well.

Read what people from around the world are saying about The Diet Fallacies!

"I thoroughly enjoyed reading this book, and I highly recommend The Diet Fallacies for anyone who needs the best in their health. The Diet Fallacies shows us how to care for the greatest asset we will ever have, our body. Al's stories get right to the point and deliver quite a bit of relevant wisdom and easy to use strategies to help embrace a healthier lifestyle. I sincerely appreciate the resource list of books, cookbooks, and movies to reinforce. Great job, I am also an advocate of the best in dietary habits, and I have no doubt you will change your life for the better when using what this powerful book has to offer."

Rich C., MD

"I am a nutritionist, and the first thing I do is encourage people to get off the junk food. This book helps you understand the addictive nature of processed garbage that is sold to us as food. It isn't food; it is carefully manipulated chemical rubbish designed to make us want to consume more, making us sick and the food companies rich."

Andie T.

"Read this book if you're ready for real change."

B.E.

"A great read with well-balanced advice for anyone. This book is factual, informative, well researched and witty."

Paresh P., UK

"Al has gotten to the gut reason why we diet and debunked it! This is a must read for yo-yo dieters and those who justify away every item they eat."

Tina B.

"Why don't diets work? What are you eating that propagates the returned weight gain once you have lost it? The Diet Fallacies takes a hard look at what we eat and why diets will not work - why they don't work. The author makes clear the addictive properties of our foods in the American way of eating. Al Davis then gives us a way of eating that will work"

Kate E.

"Coming from someone who suffered from addictions and has spent years researching food, Al Davis has put both his knowledge and his passion into this book. Don't miss the opportunity to read this book and benefit from his expertise"

Consolata D.

"This is a great book if you want to get the low-down on the misconceptions of dieting."

Colleen C., Belfast, Ireland

"Al's book speaks the truth, the hard truth about food, and the myths wrapped around it. Read it if you dare, because the truth of it will set you free!"

Alan J.

"Al Davis provides scientific support, real life examples and plenty of resources to broaden your learning so that you can decide for yourself."

Orna G.

"The information presented by Mr. Davis is so understandable, so relatable, and so undeniable that I can no longer ignore the fact that I have been putting more poison into my mouth than nutrients"

Robin R.

"Not another diet book! Fortunately, this isn't another diet, but the author unpicks the theory and practice of all the popular diets out there and explains why they don't work. The personal touches and stories make this book more than just a review of the fallacies; it makes it real because someone else has struggled and suffered through these diets."

Susan J., Australia

"This book makes me want to rethink my eating habits. If you're interested in your health, buy [it]."

Wendy H.

"Mr. Davis' style is direct and at times in your face. But that's exactly how it needs to be. He delivers his message with strength and authority. Whether you end up becoming a vegan or not, it will challenge your thinking about health and well being and the effect of what you put in your mouth. Plus, it's a damn good read."

Heather H., Australia

"Throughout the book, Mr. Davis makes you think instead of accepting given information. The book is very well put together. It is an easy read that brings you a lot of great information."

Otakara K.

"He's given me some great modification ideas on the way to eat and why. I'll definitely be utilizing my new knowledge going forward. One of my goals is to reach a healthier level of fitness in my retirement and with Al's recommendations, I know I can get there!"

Cheryl F.

"In his book based on extensive personal experience and research, Al helps us see why traditional diets are as likely to succeed as the solemn promise an alcoholic makes the morning after a bad hangover."

Hema S., Bangalore India

"I believe if we adopt the right mindsets and principles shared in this book, our desired wellness goals are not too far-fetched. This book is definitely a keeper for my library."

June L., Singapore

"Al delivers - as he shares his own struggles with over eating and the health risks he encountered, while showing every reader that victory is possible for you too! Al makes this book quite palatable as he shares his impressive research seasoned with humor!"

Susan W.

"Diet Fallacies presents the rationale for failed fad diets and offers great sound advice to simplify and successfully overcome food addictions and/or weight loss difficulties. He shares openly his experiences and struggles that led him to establishing simple guidelines and habits that work...Way to go, Mr. Davis"

Virginia R.

Table of Contents

Dedication

We are all heirs to the accumulated knowledge of the past, and hopefully the wisdom as well, whether we realize it or not. I am certainly no exception, and as it has often been stated by others, "I stand on the shoulders of giants."

I now find myself uncomfortably in the position of the many authors who write the dedication to their books, beginning with "I have so many people to thank, it is impossible to know where to start," or some variation on that theme. Nevertheless, I'll try and it can only be incomplete.

This is dedicated to my father, who taught me the value of reading and writing; to my mother, who always enjoined me to look after the needs of others; to my many, many teachers and friends in school, and those who I associated with in the rest of my life who influenced me in positive ways—and that wasn't by any means all of them!

This is also dedicated to the terrific people in Self-Publishing School, without whose influence and support, this book would not have ever been written. Particular thanks go to Chandler Bolt, Sean Summer, my coach Angie Mroczka, my partner in crime Otakara Klettke, and the many people who responded to my requests for help and advice.

Most particularly, this is dedicated to those special teachers and friends—and you know who you are—without whose help and influence my life would have stagnated, and perhaps even literally ended a number of years ago. You have helped me to begin to realize that literally none of us has any idea of what—and in which direction—our real possibilities may be. I thank each of you from the bottom of my heart.

—Al Davis, Belmont MA, 2016

Introduction & Free Offer

To readers of this book (even if you are just reading a preview on Amazon), I am also offering, absolutely free of charge, five easy to make, delicious whole foods plant based recipes!

You'll get recipes for the following: the infamous Carrot Cake Smoothie, no-cook lower fat peanut sauce, spicy pepper and tomato salsa, wild rice mélange, and a delicious granola with no added fat.

Simply go to http://curbthosecravings.com/five-free-recipes to get your download. 100% free for you.

But let's get on with the book...

The clerk looked at me indifferently as I bought the pound of M&Ms, but my attitude toward the candy was anything BUT indifferent. As I carefully bit and tore open the package (these packages explode and scatter candy everywhere if you don't, as I once found out), and quickly devoured the first mouthful, I experienced the now-familiar simultaneous pleasure, joy and rush of the first taste and sugar sensation, coupled with the instantaneous compulsion to keep shoveling them into my mouth.

Eating as I walked down 9th Street in San Francisco toward my store on Howard, I couldn't understand why this was happening. It made absolutely no sense that I should be eating this stuff by the pound. It was insane that I was packing on pounds, eating sweets until I felt sick, until my heart was throbbing madly—and not in the healthy way like after strenuous exercise, but in a scary way—and then doing it again and again, either with more candy, or ice cream, or something else sweet.

I didn't know this was directly related to something I thought I'd conquered, or at least had gotten a pretty good grip on a couple of years prior: alcohol addiction. Scientists have proved through vigorous research that alcoholics are more prone to sugar addiction because of the chemical similarities in the two. I also suspect the predisposition to compulsive and addictive behavior doesn't help either.

This stuff had me hooked and I began to overeat other things as well: pizza, sandwiches, hamburgers, and more unhealthy stuff. The weight really piled on. I knew something was happening, but I didn't know what. I didn't know at the time that white flour also has a similar addictive effect on people, creating similar irresistible cravings.

It was so close to what had happened to me with alcohol that I sought others who had the same difficulty, and pretty quickly wound up in Overeaters Anonymous. This was after trying many times, unsuccessfully, to stay away from sugar and white flour. This was from overeating and experiencing the same frustration everyone feels when they try this without knowing what they are up against.

OA only lasted a few weeks but seemed to work. However, it seemed like a rehash of what I'd learned in AA, which was fine, except that I had my own issues with the philosophy, and didn't want any more of it at that point in my life. Pretty soon after my brief association with it ended, I was gorging myself again.

Fortunately for me, I had made a connection with a company in San Francisco called <u>Stop for Life</u> (no longer in business), which I'd used to help me stop smoking, and the owner had also gotten into the weight control business. With help from him and his program, I was finally able to put the genie of overeating back into the bottle, where it has stayed for nearly 40 years.

Since then, I have been able to stay with this particular eating plan, occasionally having some sugar, but never going back to where I started. My weight stayed more or less under control because of the way I was eating. Other factors in my life helped me. My job required a lot of physical activity and I took up karate. I also put myself through a hard workout several times a week. It never occurred to me that the food I was eating was only <u>somewhat</u> healthy, not totally healthy.

As far as I was concerned, moderation was the key to good health. I figured eating some meat and cheese, with lots of fruit and veggies was key, so long as it wasn't in excess. After all, isn't that the popular wisdom, moderation in all?

And later, an 11 year marriage to a woman who was a gourmet cook didn't cause too much of a problem with my weight. My intake of meat, fish, cheese, butter and cream spiked, while my fruit and veggie intake decreased. But the work I was doing was pretty physical, and the extra calories got burned off.

Another life-changing event happened a couple of years after my second divorce (the drinking was the cause of the first divorce, years prior). I was awakened late one night by a feeling of pressure in my chest. My first thought was that I was having a heart attack, but my idea of a heart attack symptom was pain in the chest, and not pressure. I later found out that I was incorrect.

And besides, it was only recently that I had been told by my doctor that the likelihood of me having a heart attack was minimal. My blood cholesterol was around 180 (as I recall rather dimly), but I do remember the doctor saying there was no cause for alarm since the LDL to HDL ratio (i.e. the ratio of bad to good cholesterol in the blood) in my case was totally OK. I took fish oil and a baby aspirin daily. My weight was fine and I exercised regularly. I did all the right stuff, so I believed. So the thought of having a heart attack had literally never occurred to me until that night. Lying down was more painful than sitting up, and I was not able to go to sleep. Finally I got smart and called 911.

(Perhaps it goes through everyone's mind about calling 911; something like "What will they think if it's a false alarm?", but it's not the right question to be asking. A better question would be: "What might happen if I DON'T call 911?" But I digress...)

I unlatched the front door in case I wasn't able to get up again (not wanting them to have to break it down), and waited. In just a few minutes, my living room was filled with a bunch of very big and rather scary looking guys asking me questions and giving me aspirin. They helped me into the ambulance and when they shaved my chest and slapped on the paddles of the defibrillator, I knew I was in trouble.

Fast forward to the hospital, lying on the gurney in the ER, watching the ceiling tiles speed by as they rolled me down the hall to the operating room, I remember thinking that this might be my last day on earth. However, due to the exceptional care delivered by Mt. Auburn Hospital in Cambridge (thanks again, everyone!), it wasn't.

I had suffered what was called a "mild" heart attack. In terms of severity and understatement, it's sort of like a "mild" poke in the eye with a sharp stick (there is no such thing). It was a game changer and a life changer for me.

After my hospitalization, I asked my cardiologist why, despite the fact that my blood numbers were thought to be OK, this had happened. He told me that even though I ate plenty of fruits and veggies, I still had a family history of heart disease. As a result of this, he explained, I was lucky to have had a heart attack at age 66 instead of in my 40s. Even he, though, didn't know that what is considered the "normal" range is an unhealthy range for cholesterol—a fact I later discovered.

I was determined that a heart attack was never going to happen to me again. I went through cardio rehab. I found out that within what is considered this "normal" range for cholesterol in the US—namely 150 to 200, fully 35% of all heart attacks occur. A quarter of them are fatal on the spot (see http://tinyurl.com/ke9hfrw). Also, a quarter of the deaths this year in the US will be from heart attacks (see http://tinyurl.com/3c5uqz5). This got my attention!

I discovered that there was a famous heart study done a number of years ago, the Framingham Heart Study. One of many things they found was that people with combined cholesterol of less than 150 were virtually heart attack proof. When I found that out, I decided that was for me. This was the plan that Dr. Caldwell Esselstyn had proposed in his famous book, <u>How to Prevent and Reverse Heart Disease</u>. This is the plan that had worked so well for not only his patients, but with only slight variation, for those of Dr. Dean Ornish, Dr. John McDougall, and others as well. This was scientifically verified, on many occasions, by other doctors, too.

So what does this have to do with weight loss? Plenty. I discovered that the same style of eating that will both stop and reverse heart disease that Drs. Esselstyn, Ornish, and others talk about will also help you to lose weight very effectively. And it will help you lose weight in a manner that works both in the short term and in the long term. Plus, it works for virtually everyone who sticks with the program.

What is this miracle eating plan? Simple. It is whole foods, plant based, without added oil—and that means no fish oil supplements either. It also means keeping processed foods to a minimum. No meat, no fish, no poultry, no dairy. With this eating plan, virtually the entire plant kingdom is my, and can be your, culinary playground, and it's huge. My last cholesterol test came back at 119, and my weight has stabilized—but as I said, weight hasn't been a problem for years.

I have been studying nutrition intensely over the years since my illness, and I have realized that eating this way is not only the way to avoid heart disease, but it is the key to successful weight loss and weight maintenance. If you are looking to end the weight loss dilemma once and for all, plus getting the added benefit of improving your health, you owe it to yourself to continue reading this book. I realize full well that whole foods, plant based eating flies in the face of what many people consider to be "food," but stick with me, despite any misgivings and trepidation you might have.

You will not go hungry. The food is extremely tasty and not at all boring. You will get ample protein (perhaps the biggest concern people have, and in fact, I address a whole chapter to this question). You will get plenty of calcium, and no doubt a whole lot more vitamins and minerals in their natural state than you get now. Constipation will become a thing of the past. If you want seconds, take seconds! This is not a plan of deprivation or of hair shirts! You will start to improve your health. Your chances of developing chronic diseases will plummet. Your type II diabetes, or your risk for it, may well become part of your past. Plus your weight will drop. And if you stick with this eating plan, it will <u>stay</u> off as well.

The body always wants to heal and it will start to do just that if you stop putting in the things that cause obesity and so much disease in the first place: processed foods, sodas, sugar substitutes, meat, cheese, fish, and so on. Also the other high calorie, mildly toxic substances that are low in nutrients that pass for food in this country, whose deleterious effect is cumulative over time.

But consider: we don't start with a clean slate. If you've been eating the Standard American Diet (a.k.a. S.A.D.), as most of us have, you've already done damage to yourself: a buildup of arterial plaque, among other things, and a propensity toward addictive eating, fueled by processed foods, that isn't going to go away. You can learn to control this addiction, but not eliminate it.

And when you get it under control through proper eating and nutrition, your extra weight will come off by itself. Again, the body wants to heal, and obesity is a symptom of a diseased body. Remove the cause of the disease and you will heal. Just ask Bill Clinton, who adopted this way of eating following his heart surgery. He lost 25 pounds or so, as well.

And, more importantly, we have attitude problems. Plus our thinking is screwed up. We are victims, among other things, of the "Tomato Effect".

Huh?

I'll explain.

Years ago in this country most people thought that tomatoes were poisonous, apparently because certain people, not knowing any better, ate them from pewter plates. The acid in the tomatoes leached out the lead, resulting in lead poisoning. Tomatoes remained largely uneaten for many, many years because of this, even after it was demonstrated that the problem was not the tomato, people refused to eat them in America, though people were eating them in Europe!

The same thing is happening today. It's been scientifically shown many times that the whole foods plant based diet is the best diet for not only health, but for weight loss. This fact is systematically ignored by most people, including medical professionals who should know better, and dismissed by others who disagree with it without verifying one way or the other. This is one example of the tomato effect and we all suffer from it to some degree.

The tomato effect can be described as the ignoring of scientific evidence when it is at odds with current treatments or theories about disease and their treatment. The expression comes from an article in the <u>Journal of the American Medical Association</u> in 1962.

The tomato effect can be summed up in two words: "yes, but..." The underlying attitude is often "No. I disagree. You are nuts. Screw you. Pass the donuts. And I refuse to entertain what you have to say." We can keep these attitudes if we so choose, but remember, this is what keeps us—and out weight-- EXACTLY where we and it are at!

We weren't born with those attitudes. They are not genetic, any more than anyone's so-called propensity to obesity or their so-called emotional eating. If we lived in another part of the world, where people ate a more normal, plant-based diet, the thought of eating large amounts of crap foods might seem equally odd. Until the food companies started advertising, that is!

Attitudes come from ideas we have. They are thoughts we've repeated, having heard them from others, that eventually we have come to believe as truth. People have attitudes towards all sorts of things: the weather, politics, sex, religion, and so on. One thing they have in common is that we weren't born with them. They are truly not our own. But we take them as our own, calling them "our thoughts, our opinions, and our feelings".

And there is another complication: crappy food is addictive. But we'll cover that later.

This is what we have to change. We all think we are open-minded, until something like this comes along which challenges this notion. What has to change is our knee-jerk, tomato effect reaction to new ideas, or at least to these new ideas I'm putting forth. If that doesn't change, we will continue to suffer, not only from the tomato effect, but the pizza effect, the hamburger effect, and the junk food effect. And the price tag will be much higher for us than just avoiding a few tomatoes.

In fact, the idea of "never dieting again" may seem equally "out there!"

Technically, this is a vegan approach, but I do not like nor do I use the word. "Vegan" doesn't mean healthy or conducive to weight loss or maintenance. It simply means eating that doesn't include any products from animals.

And so by that definition, potato chips and Oreos are vegan. And there are plenty of vegans who are quite overweight. Go to any vegan group gathering or vegetarian restaurant and you will see what I mean.

Also, this is not a political approach. I won't be suggesting that anyone not eat honey because it exploits honeybees, nor will I be telling people to avoid leather because it comes from animals. If anybody wants to stay away from these things, it's their business, not mine. Avoiding animal products is a great way to do our part in reversing global warming since something like 51% of greenhouse gas emission is due to factory farming (the number varies depending on the source, but it is always high); but that isn't the thrust of this book either. And by taking the whole foods plant based approach, fewer animals will be subject to lives of unbelievable cruelty, but this is the last time I'll be mentioning this.

This book is not about getting someone to be able to fit into a size seven, or for the guys, to make us a ripped super stud with a six pack. If that happens, great, but it's not the focus.

If somebody wants to be a sex object, or impress his buddies, that's his or her business, not mine.

You will notice that there may appear to be a certain amount of repetition in this book, and in the approach of presenting ideas. If that seems to be the case, I stand guilty as charged. Many ideas in here are probably new and unfamiliar to you, and by presenting them more than once, and from slightly different angles each time, they hopefully will be more familiar and therefore more approachable.

This is also an approach to weight loss where judgment of ourselves, or others, isn't a helpful part of the process. At least as much as possible, since we all judge ourselves and each other to one degree or the other (would you want to take weight loss advice from someone who weighed 300 pounds? I didn't think so!). There is no profit in judging others for what they eat or don't eat, plant based or otherwise, and there is no profit in judging ourselves for our shortcomings, real or imagined, either. So please try to avoid it, as much as possible—and I realize this is a tall order!

(And I am sure some people will realize that they have become like me, judging myself for judging myself. But I digress...)

You will find, though, that as the weight starts coming off, your self-judgment will begin to diminish. After all, can you judge yourself for being overweight if you no longer are? And that's just the beginning of the good things that will start to unfold in your private, inner world.

You are very fortunate. You have the key in your hand in the form of this book to an adventure in eating, in health, and in living a new and transformed life. But like any key, you need to use it. You have to stick it in the lock and turn it. Then you have to open the door, walk through it, and stay on the other side.

It is a process, not an instant fix. **There are none**. It takes effort and sometimes it's tough. It takes time. This plan I present isn't about just losing weight, it's about helping you change your relationship to food and your lifestyle. We need to re-learn how to eat. We've spent years getting our problem to where it is right now, and although it may not take as much time to get back to where we should or want to be, it's still a process that does take time. For some, it will take more time; for some less.

But it is SOOO worth it! So please continue with this book and this plan. It is written with the hard-learned lessons, the work, and pain of many people, not just me, and is delivered to you with my love and wishes for your success and health for the rest of your life.

Al Davis
Belmont MA
2016
www.CurbThoseCravings.com

1. The Scope of the Problem
(Or, How'd we all get so BIG?)

There is an idea about invisibility—not my idea, but one that goes like this: Certain things are invisible because that is in their very nature. For example, ideas, thoughts and emotions are invisible. Certain things are invisible because they are too small—like microbes, atoms, molecules, and so on. Certain things are invisible because they are too large—the earth, for example—we simply cannot get a sense of it from our vantage point. Certain things are invisible because they are too distant, such as stars and distant galaxies. Certain things are invisible because they are ubiquitous, for example the overt racism of fifty or a hundred years ago was largely invisible to most white people. And the less overt racism of today still is, for the most part—at least if you are white.

There is the "out of sight, out of mind" sort of invisibility, for example, the many, many people who rarely, if ever, appear in public: war veterans in the VA; the people who have lost a limb or their eyesight through type II diabetes, a condition which is generally both preventable and reversible; those whose deteriorated health or massive obesity keeps them confined to their home or to a care facility of some kind; or those who are so ashamed of how they look because they are so heavy that they rarely go out.

And certain things are invisible because we unquestioningly take them as reality.

This last type of invisibility will be one of the subjects of this book. Obesity, the fallacy of diets, and the concomitant health care crisis as a result primarily of the foods we eat are damaging and destroying us individually to greater or lesser degrees, and show absolutely no signs of diminishing or abating using the current methods. And for the most part, these causes are totally invisible to us—medical professionals as well as lay people—until we begin to take the blinders off.

Imagine a time many years ago, in a more innocent age, where there was no Internet, phones had cords and live operators, TV shows were still in black and white, and people ate meat and cheese without a second thought. This was also a time when there were cigarette ads in on TV and in magazines, doctors smoked cigarettes during appointments—and actually recommended them for weight loss and to help people to relax—and lung cancer deaths were, not surprisingly, on the rise.

Then the Surgeon General's report came onto the scene in 1964, and we all know what happened as a result of that: smoking rates dropped dramatically, as did the lung cancer rate. And there was a huge amount of pushback, not only from the consumers, but from cigarette manufacturers as well.

We are in a similar age right now. Only the faint glimmerings of public awareness are becoming evident now, but we are in the midst of what is called a "health care crisis," brought on primarily by the foods we eat, promulgated by industry, assisted by government, and even encouraged by the very doctors who should know better, who write out prescriptions, and then go have a hamburger for lunch. And this is as invisible to us as the problem of cigarettes was invisible to all but the tobacco companies, and a few more perceptive people.

Plus, we are surrounded by food. We have food temptations undreamt of in known history, not by the mightiest or wealthiest king. And these temptations are available 24-7 to all of us, via either our being surrounded by it at home, or by ads on TV, in movies, or on the internet—and they can be delivered to the peace and comfort of your home.

And what passes for food isn't really what used to be known as food at all. It's mostly processed. It's loaded with sugar, salt and fat, in proportions and ratios and in portion sizes designed so that we can't stop eating, and so that we keep coming back for more. For the most part, we do not see the truth of this. We do not allow the truth to set us free from the food that is not only a major contributor to weight gain, but which—with its high calorie and sodium content and low nutrient value—is inherently unhealthy as well, and which eventually leads to disease: the so-called "health care crisis".

But invisibility isn't the only problem with the obesity dilemma most of us face; the whole arena is filled with fallacy as to the nature of the problem and what to do about it. And of course, no one agrees as to what is correct and what isn't. So don't be surprised if you find yourself disagreeing with some of what is said in this book. I do encourage you to keep reading, despite disagreement, since your disagreement is coming from how you think right now— and how you think right now is what got you into the situation you are now in. And your situation and weight aren't going to change until your thinking changes.

(I assume you want to change your situation and your weight, don't you?)

The media are constantly asking questions such as whether someone you know or love has been affected by alcoholism/drug addiction/violence/suicide (choose one). But when is the last time you were ever asked the question as to whether someone's life was affected by obesity, addictive overeating, or illness and death as a result of poor food choices? Do you think a death certificate ever lists obesity or poor food choices as a cause of death?

Probably rarely if ever. Poor food choices are not seen as causal to the myriad of personal and social problems that they do cause; they are totally invisible in the grand scheme of things. You are never going to be asked this question about whether anyone you know or love has been affected by poor eating choices, simply because the problem is mostly invisible. No one sees food choices as the cause of so many personal and social problems. And they are behind a HUGE percentage of our health problems.

If an illegal drug of some kind came out that did to us—and to as many of us—what we do willingly to ourselves through diet, we would be outraged, everyone would support efforts to neutralize this threat to our nation, and perhaps something might be done. Or if terrorists killed 600,000 people a year as heart attacks do, the nation would mobilize immediately. But the government itself is partially responsible for this crisis, despite wars on obesity, food pyramids, and so on. So the problem remains below the radar, from this point of view, it remains invisible.

And most people have no idea of how they have been seduced into addiction to foods that get them fat, destroy their health bit by bit, and cause us to pass this curse on to our children. Again, it's an invisible problem. And in fact, a problem that many if not most people would deny even exists at all.

But ultimately, once we've seen this problem as it is and for what it is, we have the power to address and to change it for ourselves, individually, and not through government intervention: through our food choices. It may be a long time—if ever—before America and the rest of the world wake up and realize what we are doing to ourselves; the government isn't going to help, and even if there is national change, it certainly won't happen quickly enough for us in our lives. So we have to do the job ourselves. First, we have to discover what the problem is. Then by finding out what poor food choices are doing—and can and will do—to us and to those we love. And then by taking on the task of moving in a different direction, to the direction of vibrant health and normal weight, not living with just the absence of symptoms or disease, which is the usual medical approach to disease.

For the fallacies of food choices, dieting, obesity and the health care crisis are as invisible as microbes and distant galaxies until we start investigating them. Diets don't work, never did work, can't work, and won't work no matter how often we try to use them. The health care crisis that is the ungodly child of poor food choices isn't going to go away until we address the cause: namely the food choices we are making in the moment. And our lives—and weight—aren't going to change until and unless we start learning what the real problem is, and applying the solution to ourselves.

For if someone considers and treats what he or she calls their weight problem as separate from the cause, they are doomed to fail. The weight will come off, on some sort of diet—as no doubt has happened before--and when that person has dropped the weight they think they need to lose, they will go off the diet. And we all know what happens after that: after a period of time, sometimes longer, sometimes shorter, the old habits start to reassert themselves, and before long they eat like they've always eaten—only probably more voraciously. And of course they wind up gaining back the weight they've lost—and then some. Sound familiar?

This new way of eating, like I say, is not pixie dust or magic wands. It does take effort. It does take time. But not as much effort as dragging around an extra 20 , 50, or 100 pounds of weight every hour of each and every day for the rest of our shortened lives. Nowhere near as much effort as constantly thinking and obsessing about food on a minute to minute basis, enduring the emotional burden of having our eating out of control, of beating ourselves up about it for the rest of our lives; not as much effort as spending time and energy having or recuperating from diseases such as a heart attack, gout, hypertension, diabetes, and so on. I could go on and on, but you get the point.

What it takes, and what is the point of difficulty for many people, is it takes change. Of doing things differently, of becoming open to new ideas, things we hadn't considered, and going in a different direction with our food and our eating.

But it's true—diets DO work for a small number of people. By varying estimates, around five percent of the people who start a diet actually keep the weight off (and there are reasons to strongly question that number). Yes, Weight Watchers does work for some people. Yes, Paleo, Zone, Atkins and so on do manage to help a number of people not only lose weight, but keep it off. But if you are reading this book, my guess is that you've tried these approaches.

This book isn't for you if you think that diets—and their infinite variations—will work for you over the long haul. If you think that doing the same thing again and again will magically yield different results, this book isn't for you. If you think there is some hidden secret, some arcane formula, that will solve your weight problem once and for all—and that all you have to do is buy the newest book, or buy the latest supplement, eat lots of meat and cheese, or avoid carbs, or eat super foods, or whatever—and all will be roses, roses—if this is your thinking, please return this book to whomever you got it from and get your money back. Otherwise you will be wasting your money.

As Hippocrates said, "Let medicine be thy food, and thy food be thy medicine".

2. Basic Tenets of this Book
(Or, A second serving of answers to the above)

So let's go. This book is centered on a group of ideas that are core to an understanding of the problem, and the solution. I've touched on or alluded to some of these a bit, but let's nail them a little more specifically.

First, that American eating habits have been taken over from the individual by the corporate, and that what we now mostly eat has corporate interests involved, instead of our health and weight interests.

Second, that American business, through food science, has discovered and implemented a type of food that is irresistible, hyper-palatable, and addictive, such that when we start eating, it's difficult if not impossible to stop, and that we have become, to one degree or another, a nation of food junkies for this type of food. This is not just junk foods, but restaurant and packaged foods, which have become staples as well.

And what has happened is, that a result of this, we have come to prefer this sort of food, so it's what we cook at home, instead of the plain, simple fare that most people ate for tens of thousands of years, which kept their weight down.

We have become used to high fat foods that are laden with sugar and salt as a part of our daily diet and, unknown to us, these are the very foods that create a mechanism called craving, which makes it impossible for most of us to limit our intake of them. Between the psychological component of familiarity and habit, and the physical mechanism of craving, once we start, we don't stop. And just one bite leads to another, which makes control impossible.

Third, that government has not only been complicit, but encouraging this, because it's good for business.

Fourth, this processed food lifestyle most of us have is the main (not the only) cause of weight gain and obesity (and the diseases of lifestyle—heart attacks, strokes, and the rest) in this country, which we are now sadly exporting to the rest of the world, with predictable results.

Fifth, the only way out of this morass—at least at this point in time—is the individual. To reclaim not only our natural weight, but our health, we need to go in a totally different direction. We need to adopt a style of eating that does not cause the cravings that the Standard American Diet (SAD, as I mentioned) does, but that still tastes really good and that we can stay with.

It's too late for us to return to the ultra-simple foods of several hundred years ago, but we can recreate our own version of it today; in fact we can have an even healthier version because of advances in the science of nutrition, and because of the availability of so many different things all year around. And it can be geared to our different tastes. Plus it is a way of eating that we can be both happy and satisfied with.

Perhaps over time the rest of the country will wake up (and there is evidence it's happening to a degree), but it hasn't happened yet.

Sixth, the only way of eating that does all this is whole foods, plant based. Yup, you heard me. Veggies, beans, grains, legumes, fruit—as has been said by others, "Nothing with a face or a mother." It's the recommended eating plan of the nation's largest health insurer, Kaiser Permanente, it's the recommended way of eating of the former President of the American College of Cardiology Kim Williams, and you'll be eating in the company of Bill Clinton, Ellen Degeneres, Lev Tolstoy, and many, many others. Do a web search for "famous vegans," if you're curious. You will meet more of these people later.

And this is not some sort of dietary hair shirt philosophy— the food is delicious! Otherwise we would all be doomed to either overeating for the rest of our overweight lives, or living off carrot and celery sticks with brown rice. Not a cheerful prospect!

I realize this seems like a radical new direction for many of you, but consider the following: If we do what everyone else is doing, from eating to dieting, we will get the same totally predictable, law conformable results that everyone else gets: obesity and ill health, with all the personal, familial, social, and business anguish that this brings on. What you are now eating, and your futile attempts to lose weight, is what you will be doing for the rest of your 100% predictable life, unless you make a shift.

Are you ready to at least consider a different direction?

3. The Diet Fallacies
(It's what we know that just ain't so!)

This is our problem, individually and collectively. The actual quote from Mark Twain is, "It ain't what you don't know that gets you into trouble. It's what you know for sure that just ain't so". But in the case of diet and weight loss, it's both what you don't know that gets you into trouble, and what you do know that is false, that does the same. We are enmeshed and ensnared in lies, errors, misinformation—and flat-out fallacies about diet and diet weight loss.

So let's go after a few of these that have affected all of us to one degree or another. There isn't just one fallacy about diet and weight loss; like I said, the whole field is rife with them. And of course, no one agrees as to what is correct and what isn't. So I'll try to separate what is fact from what is clearly opinion—or out and out nonsense.

Let's start with the biggest myth about obesity, being overweight, and dieting. Are you ready?

We read headlines and we hear TV. We hear public figures screaming about the "obesity epidemic" and how over 2/3 of the people in this country are either obese or overweight. You also hear how one in three kids and teens is overweight. And we even have fat cats and dogs! What happens, of course—and unfortunately—is that we hear it so often it fails to shock us anymore.

Here's the kicker. Obesity is NOT the problem. Being overweight is NOT the problem.

Huh?

"Al, do you mean to tell me that if I am a hundred pounds overweight, that isn't the problem?"

Nope. It's simply not the problem. Period. It's A problem. And it is a really BIG problem. But it isn't THE problem. How's THAT for a new idea? How is THAT for a different way of thinking?

Here's the deal: weight is the SYMPTOM of the problem. Weight is the EFFECT of the problem.

I'll give you some examples, which will help explain what I mean. If sea levels are rising because of global warming melting the ice caps, is the solution to the problem to build sea walls? It may be a necessary stopgap measure, but it's definitely not a solution to the problem.

If a smoker is coughing and hacking, is the solution to his problem to get him some medicated lozenges? Of course not—but smokers do this anyway—(I know, 'cause I used to use lozenges when I smoked).

If you knew a guy who was a heavy drinker, who regularly parked his car on his neighbor's front lawn, who ran over pedestrians, had car crashes, spun donuts in the park, and who could never find his car the next morning after drinking you probably have some sort of idea what this guy's problem is, don't you?

Would you suggest he get some sort of GPS locator for his car? That he take driving lessons? That he get more insurance?

NO, OF COURSE NOT!!! That would be DUMB! The problem is that the guy has a drinking problem. The drinking is the CAUSE of all that follows. The crashes and all the rest of it are the EFFECT of the drinking.

But if you were twenty, fifty, or a hundred pounds overweight, and you went to the doctor, you might get diagnosed with high blood pressure, high cholesterol, type II diabetes, diverticulitis, constipation, and a whole bunch of other fun things, and what does the doctor do? He or she gives you a prescription for pills to take for the symptoms. And in a "By the way", tells you to lose weight. By eating less of what you already eat, or to cut back. To try to eat "moderately," those things which can't be eaten moderately, and which cause all the problems in the first place, does not and cannot work.

The two of you are unwittingly performing a dance that's repeated constantly around the country, with only one possible outcome: the prompt—or at least the eventual—return to "business as usual".

So let's look a bit more at the fallacy of dieting. And I'm going to use another ridiculous example to make the point. Remember the movie "Supersize Me"? If you haven't seen it, go see it. This guy tried living off MacDonald's "food" for an extended period of time. He wound up getting sick. His blood tests were a disaster. He gained a whole lot of weight. Would you or any other reasonably sane person argue that the solution to his problem is that he should go to a doctor for pills? That he has a weight problem? NO, OF COURSE NOT! He got sick and fat because of the stuff he was putting down his throat and because of his commitment to doing it to make this movie! The solution isn't to start popping pills—it's to start eating healthy foods again, and the body will heal itself.

Sadly, we are all victims of the same sort of thinking, although it is generally harder to see when it concerns us personally. When we think of dieting, we think of trying to address an effect. We are NOT addressing the <u>cause</u> of the problem. The problem is simple and obvious when you think about it a bit differently—it's our EATING, and our thoughts and feelings about eating, plus our habits around eating. The effect is the weight. The weight isn't the problem; it's the effect of the problem. The weight doesn't just show up. Some things may just happen, (like the bumper sticker says) but weight has a definite cause.

The human body is incredibly self regulating—and fortunately for us, as I said, self-healing if given the right circumstances. Billions of things are happening, all day, all night, totally invisibly to us (there's that word again). We breathe, all day and all night long. If we exert ourselves, the body knows how much more oxygen we need, and starts us breathing more heavily until we re-oxygenate ourselves. If we are thirsty, we'll drink water until we've had enough. People don't usually hyperventilate or drink too much water. The body self-regulates both oxygen and water intake by telling you when to stop.

And believe it or not, your body can be trained—or better, can re-learn—to do the same thing with food. There is a built-in "stop" mechanism when our body senses we've had enough food. It's not a thought. It's a simple, quiet sensation of "I've had enough." We stop eating when we've had enough in the same way we only breathe what we need or drink water to sate our thirst. But—and this is a BIG but, we have to give it the right food and the right circumstances to work with.

We just didn't happen out of the blue in the past twenty or thirty years to start eating in a way that got us to where we are today, though. There aren't any fat genes, which suddenly showed up on the scene. We can't blame them!

The change was progressive, like any addiction, and it's more like this—and what I am about to tell you here is but the tip of a very big iceberg, so I will summarize.

The processed foods most people eat today have been engineered to bypass that "stop" mechanism that we all have naturally. It's stated quite explicitly in that Lay's Potato Chip ad, "Bet you can't eat just one." Certain combinations of ingredients, centered on sugar, salt and fat, create cravings that are ***addictively irresistible***. They work with pleasure centers in the brain by hyper-stimulation, by affecting them intensely, and in ways not found in nature, in the same way that narcotics do, and create a similar craving and addiction.

Entire industries of consultants and scientists work in conjunction with the food industry to create, test, and market this stuff to us. You wonder why it's so hard to stop eating junk? This is why! It's really rather frightening, when the truth of this begins to dawn on you, how big, how all pervasive, and how totally invisible the problem is.

The food industry tries to get us to increase our intake of foods that are inherently addictive, but then tells us to maintain a healthy weight by a reduced intake. Ha! In the same way an alcoholic can't limit his intake of booze after taking the first drink, it's likewise impossible for most people, once they've passed a certain point of becoming accustomed to these substances, to limit their intake of processed foods. Don't believe me? Look at the record with food. YOUR record. Right or wrong?

What would you say to a liquor ad that told alcoholics to limit their intake so as not to get drunk? Makes no sense, does it? What about a cigarette ad that told people to limit themselves to one or two a day? But we don't recognize food as a similar and equally pernicious addiction. Food addiction is largely invisible, except to the person caught up in it. And, here's the kicker: it's socially acceptable.

There is the other problem that's connected with this. That's the fact, like I said, that we unconsciously try to recreate this same sort of eating experience when we cook at home. We've acquired a taste for this sort of food. We use lots of sugar, salt and fat when we make meals. We keep using the very things that cause the problems in the first place. So we have the double whammy of processed foods, plus unhealthy and fat-causing foods we make ourselves—if indeed we do actually cook at home.

So is it surprising that we are also in the middle of a "health care crisis"? Where the healthcare system is getting so swamped, that we are spending more and more on healthcare, and medications, and so on—and still getting sicker—but again, this isn't the problem. The real problem is that we are poisoning ourselves with the foods we are eating and overeating, and thinking the problem is the health care system, rather than our individual responsibility.

Is it realistic to constantly bombard our bodies with processed foods—or even homemade foods—that are low in nutrients, high in calories, and filled with chemicals, and not expect there to be consequences—like weight gain and disease? Hardly!

You can do your own personal part to end the health care crisis by changing what you eat. As I have been trying to drive home, the solution is the whole foods, plant based diet. It's delicious, nutritious, filling, and infinitely varied. For there is no point to living to a ripe, old age if you are living to a ripe, pill-popping, sick old age—at least in my opinion! As far as I am concerned, if I am going to live to a ripe old age, I want to be well fed and healthy to the end—don't you?

Here's another fallacy for you to consider, namely that you have to eat mostly certain foods to make you lose weight faster. Well, here's another myth that sold books, I suppose. Celery, cabbage, broccoli, and other low calorie foods were promoted as things to eat to help you lose weight quicker. Usually they are high water content foods that are also low in calories, the idea being to fill you up so you aren't hungry, or that there are magical super-foods that will drop pounds without effort.

There are a few problems with this approach. First, nobody wants to—or ever will—eat celery and cucumbers or expensive super-foods all the time. Those are great, but all the time? And we've probably tried it before—I know I have. It maybe lasts a day or two, and then it starts to drive us nuts. Or for nuts, as the case may be. Plus it focuses on weight, and not lifestyle. And changing weight and lifestyle takes effort.

The only way to lose weight—and keep it off—is by eating in a satisfying, filling, and nutritionally balanced way. Not by focusing on some very limited aspect of a very large food spectrum. Or super-foods, sold to you by someone with a profit motive.

Here's another fallacy that makes the rounds: you have to exercise constantly to lose weight and to keep it off.

Well, it's one of these myths that has a bit of truth to it, as most of them do, but upon investigation, we find it's just that: a partial truth. It is of course based on the fallacy that weight is the problem—as are other myths—but let's dig deeper.

Let's attack this one in the following manner—by using an extreme example. Let's say you went on a starvation diet or became a "breatharian." You ate no food at all, nothing. No vitamins, no juices, nothing but water. Would you lose weight? Sure you would. Did you need to exercise in order to lose this weight? Quite the opposite—you'd wind up so exhausted from lack of calories and nutrition that you probably wouldn't be able to do much of anything until you finally died from starvation. And you would have lost a bunch of weight without exercising.

This is NOT the recommended way to lose weight, by the way. It's using an extreme example to make a point.

Let's say you want to take an intelligent approach and to totally change your eating habits and patterns. Do you have to exercise in order for the weight loss process to happen, as well as for the weight to come off? The short answer is no. The longer answer is twofold. One, it will help, and two, you will have more energy than you've had in years, and unless you aren't able to do exercise for some reason, you will probably want to anyway!

While it is certainly true that many more of us are exercising much less, and are much more sedentary than we once were, lack of exercise is only a minor part of the problem

But let's introduce something here again by illustrating a concept. This is not 100% scientifically accurate and is more tongue in cheek than anything, but it demonstrates a point—the Law of the Fortune Cookie. What—you've never heard of the Law of the Fortune Cookie?

The concept is as follows. Imagine after a Chinese meal in a restaurant, you get a fortune cookie. Made of white flour, white sugar, vanilla, maybe a bit of sesame oil; each has about 30 calories. Not a lot, that's for sure. Not exactly a health food either, that's also for sure. We usually don't even think of the calories when we eat them—or not.

Now, in order to gain a pound, it is generally considered that you need to take in around 3500 calories over what your body needs to maintain its current weight. And yes, I know, there are other opinions on this—I'm using this to make a point. Let's assume we are neither gaining nor losing weight, our body is at stasis.

We eat one little 30 calorie fortune cookie a day for a year. Or an additional 30 calories of anything else, for that matter. We've taken in 10,950 extra calories over what our body needs, in this year, since we were originally at the point when we were neither gaining nor losing. Dividing that by 3500, it means we've gained 3.128 pounds over the course of that year. Not too much you say? After ten years, you've gained over 31 pounds just by eating an extra 30 calories a day. A LOUSY 30 calories a day!

Let's again say your weight is at stasis, at equilibrium. Let's say you start drinking a latte a day from Starbucks. Five days a week, whole milk, for a year. There are 190 calories in a tall latte—that's almost 50 calories more than in a can of Coke, by the way—and add a teaspoon of sugar—16 calories, that makes a total of 206 calories. Do this five days in a week and it is 950 calories. Multiply that by 52 weeks in the year (you drink coffee on vacation, don't you?). That's a whopping 49,400 extra calories a year you are taking in. Which translates to 14.11 pounds you've just added this year by drinking only one latte a day over your caloric needs. Multiply this by ten, and you see where this is heading. Nowhere you want to go, that's for sure!

"A latte a day, and your tummy will pay." (And you can quote me!)

So let's make this law work in our favor. In the same way, just as 30 calories a day extra will make us gain just over 3 pounds a year, 30 calories a day LESS than we need will drop just over 3 pounds a year. Yes, I know you want to drop weight faster than that, but hear me out.

Exercise will do the same thing. If you just do a bit of walking each day—moderate pace, no death marches—and so on—it takes approximately 20 minutes to burn up a hundred calories. Obviously exact results depend on your size, but I'm illustrating a principle here. That's a thousand calories over five days. That's 18,980 calories in a year. And that's nearly five and a half pounds you've lost (or haven't gained) because you've just taken a short walk five days a week. And you can do this in a mall, if you want, as long as you don't pause to window shop.

Obviously, check with your doctor if you have any question at all if this is right for you, though.

If you look up WebMD (www.webmd.com), you can get a pretty good idea of what your caloric needs are. It's not rocket science—if you eat more than that, you gain weight, if you eat less, you lose weight. But how do you eat less than that without starving yourself and driving yourself batty?

As a hint, after you start eating the healthy foods your body really needs, you will probably find you have a whole lot more energy than you used to, and exercise is a great thing to do with all that energy.

The answer to the question of whether you need to exercise to lose weight and maintain weight loss is: no, you don't, but it helps and you will probably want to!

By the way, and this is a very big "by the way," both the government and the big food companies, in their incestuous in-cahoots sort of way, have mounted an argument that the obesity problem is due to our sedentary lifestyle and lack of exercise. Since the government and the food companies are totally in bed with each other in perpetuating the status quo of feeding us the foods that cause the problems in the first place, it's not a surprising thing to hear. It's called "blame the victim," which is like blaming a woman for enticing a man to rape her.

It's also sort of like blaming the lack of literacy of kids from lower socioeconomic areas solely on the children involved, rather than on the lousy school systems and the attitudes of the power structure toward certain groups of people.

4. The Carbohydrate Fallacy
(Or, Eat the damn things, already!)

You can't go into a grocery store today without seeing "low carb" on labels everywhere: on bread, on crackers, on cookies, and on pretty much everything else. I even saw a low carb label on 100% beef Bubba Burgers! "Low carb" is another of the bills of goods that has been sold to us under the umbrella fallacy of weight loss being a good thing. So let's look at this low carb sub-fallacy, if you will, to find out what is really going on.

As I mentioned earlier, the whole notion of dieting focuses on the wrong thing: weight loss.

Not only are these diets focused on the wrong thing, but low carb diets are often inducing an unnatural or unhealthy state in order to force the weight loss: ketosis, starvation, or attempting to control the uncontrollable; the addiction. And since the body just wants to get back to normal, to stasis and to health (except in the case of addiction), the body will resist and thwart your every attempt.

There are a number of low carb diets out there, so let's speak in the most general terms about them, since the principles apply across the board.

The most famous one is the Atkins diet, with a few subsequent spinoffs, and this bit of insanity wants people to eat a "high animal protein, low carb" diet, for the purpose of losing weight. Great, if weight was the problem—which I've already talked about—but it's not. And there are a few more problems with this as well—which I am only going to briefly touch on: the cholesterol in the meat and the cheese.

The higher your blood cholesterol gets the greater your risk of heart disease, and a whole host of other cheery things. Do you really think that by packing in the steak, chicken, bacon and pork you won't be inviting a heart attack? And meat protein—not just the cholesterol—has its own problems as well. But now even the government is telling us to limit our consumption of meat, and telling us that bacon is a carcinogen. Plus, it's been well documented that meat consumption increases the risk of colon cancer.

Second is the lack of carbs. To suggest that we get rid of carbs because they are causing us to be fat is like suggesting that we cut off our heads to keep our hair from growing grey or falling out as we get older. The body is designed to run on carbs.

People have been surviving mostly on carbs for most of human existence. Wheat, rice, potatoes, and whole grains of many kinds have been staples in the human diet. Entire civilizations were founded, maintained, and ultimately met their demise with a diet consisting primarily of carbohydrates. It also gave them all the protein they needed. People simply couldn't afford the food we eat on a meal-by-meal, day to day basis. Things like meat and cheese were the food of kings, and were eaten by the commoners only on holidays. And it was kings and nobility that suffered from the "diseases of kings". Remember Henry VIII? Not exactly the picture of health!

And most people today don't distinguish between whole grain carbs and processed ones. The problem is that we generally feed ourselves the PROCESSED carbs: the white flour, the white rice, white sugar, and so on. Processed carbs are a big problem, but whole grains most definitely are not. I'll go into this a lot more later, there is a TON of scientific evidence to back this up, but it is the TYPE of carb that is the problem, not the carb itself.

Carbohydrates are the basic fuel for the human mechanism, and to get rid of them is just silly. It's like trying to run a car on the wrong type of gasoline, it may work for a while, but eventually, there will be mechanical problems and it will break down.

Do you think people would carbo-load, just prior to running marathons, if they didn't realize at least at some level, that carbs are what gives you better endurance?

Ever hear of steak-loading prior to a marathon? I didn't think so.

Third, the lack of a balance of fruit and vegetables. Let's look at it briefly from a couple of different points of view. Health depends on eating a variety of food, not just steak and potatoes. or peanut butter and jelly. We need a variety. There is a veritable cornucopia of health and nutrition awaiting you in the world of fruits and vegetables, and to ignore the bulk of it, as the low carb people seem to want you to do, is to ignore that which will get and keep you healthy. We need diversity in our diet, not just meat and cheese.

Not to mention also that these whole fruits and vegetables provide something that the Atkins diet provides very little of: fiber. This is the stuff that keeps things moving in the digestive tract, among other things, and that, by the way, can help prevent colon cancer.

Do you think that someone, having undergone a colostomy, and changing the bag that's attached to their side, will be thinking, "All those steaks and bacon were totally worth it?" Would you be thinking that? And that's only assuming you even survive!

Perhaps if I haven't convinced the reader that being overweight is an effect, that the problem is their eating and what they eat, and if they don't mind spiking their cholesterol, depriving themselves nutritionally and subjecting themselves to the risks of eating huge amounts of meat, and plugging their intestines and colon up so badly that they'll need to call Roto-Rooter, the Atkins diet will be right up their alley.

(By the way, Dr. Atkins was overweight himself and had heart disease. Would you buy, or follow, a diet plan from an overweight guy with heart problems caused by diet? I hope not!)

This is a very brief overview on a big topic and I've hit some of the high points. Hopefully you've begun to suspect or to realize that carbs are not the problem. To say that carbs are all bad or the whole problem is like saying that all food is bad because food makes you gain weight. That's simply not the case. There's much more to it than that.

Don't just take my word for it, though. There are plenty of books and videos listed in the "resources" section, many written by medical doctors. Check those out. And come to your own conclusions.

Next in our list of diet fallacies is that, in order to maintain any weight loss I have achieved, I need to control my intake of certain foods. This is another one that's partially true. But here's the kicker: there are some foods you can control your consumption of, and some with which that's not possible.

Can you control how much you eat of sugary treats? Pizza? Ice Cream? Oreos? Potato chips or Fritos? I didn't think so. I can't either! What would you think, knowing what you now know, of a weight maintenance plan that told you to limit yourself to a half a donut every three days, a slice of pizza once a week, a half cup of ice cream every two weeks, and a cup of potato chips as a Saturday snack? How long do you think it would take before you started eating next week's allotment this week, or eating three quarters of a cup of ice cream since the container was practically empty, and so on? If you are anything like me, it wouldn't be long at all.

This stuff—this processed food—and I'm not just talking about the total junk like this, I'm also talking about the things like frozen dinners, frozen entrees, vegetables with sauce, frozen or packaged macaroni and cheese, bottled sodas and juices, and so on—all the stuff made with huge amounts of sugar, salt and fat—triggers the addictive reaction in us, as we saw earlier.

And often you don't even know the sugar, salt and fat are there and that they're having an effect on you! What happens then is that we find ourselves literally unable to stop once we start. So the question of eating this stuff moderately becomes impossible.

In AA, they tell you that it's the first drink that does it, but that's not quite accurate. And it's not even the first SIP that does it, although that's closer to what's really happening. The thing that starts the alcoholic drinking again is the DECISION to drink. It's something inside of us, something in us throws its weight. It's not the booze. It's not the nagging wife, or husband, the job loss, the death in the family, or any other stuff that people lie to themselves about. We say, "Screw it", and we are off and running.

The same thing is true of maintaining a healthy eating plan. If someone decides to go "off the wagon," so to speak, it's a DECISION. And it's THEIR decision, that THEY made, and THEY will be the one to pay.

Again, what would you think of a program for alcoholics that told them to limit themselves to one drink a week or a stop smoking plan that limited people to one cigarette a week? You would think—and with good reason—"What's with these morons that are coming up with this stuff?" And yes, I know there are exceptions to this, there may be a small number of people who seem to have an addiction under control, and you know what? Like I said earlier, if you were that exception, you wouldn't be reading this right now, I assure you.

This, by the way, is the part of the fallacy of the "cheat" day, which I will treat in Chapter 16.

If you think I am exaggerating on this point about the craving mechanism and addictive eating, please look at your personal track record and then tell me what's happening both with you and in this country. Again, there is a huge amount of misinformation, lies and other propaganda out there, and this, coupled with the self-deception we all allow ourselves—myself included—keeps us right where we are. If we want to get off this enlarging and expanding treadmill, we need to go in a totally different direction. Period.

So let's debunk yet another fallacy that may be rearing its ugly head right about now. That "experts," from the doctor, to the FDA to your neighbor or co-workers, know what they are talking about when it comes to diet, nutrition and weight loss.

Or, more importantly, those same "experts" in the inner world of our private thoughts and feelings that are right now objecting to what I am saying, because the voice of familiarity is more trusted and less threatening to the status quo than what I'm saying.

Other than our internal "experts," there are countless examples in history of where the so-called "experts" of the world have later been proven to be totally wrong, to have been leading us down a dangerous path.

Let's go back to the father of medicine, Hippocrates. He lived in a time when most people thought that the gods controlled everything. That invisible forces that we knew of but couldn't see controlled all aspects of our lives, including disease. So when we got sick, it was pretty apparent that we had done something to displease one of the gods.

Hippocrates was a revolutionary in his time. He proposed that wasn't the case, that there were other things going on and that disease had nothing to do with the gods. Do you think this idea was well received back in ancient Greece? Or do you think, more likely, that he got the same sort of kickback from others that any new idea—true or not—always gets?

Moving forward in history, let's go back only a few hundred years to the time of Galileo, around 1600, where it was generally considered by all the experts (and yes, I know, there are many different versions of this; please seek the point I am making, rather than pecking the argument apart), all the assembled geniuses of the church in Italy, and anywhere else within their sphere of influence, that the sun revolved around the earth. Galileo professed to the world that the Earth did indeed revolve around the Sun, going against the "experts" in Rome. In 1615, during one of the Inquisitions, Galileo was arrested and forced to recant his statement, pleading guilty in court for lying and sentenced to house arrest for life. Let's hear it for the experts.

It was also once thought that the Earth was flat, that if you sailed too far in one direction, to the land portrayed as being populated by dragons and sea monsters on old maps, you would simply fall off. Apparently no one ever wondered why all the water in the ocean never drained away, but that seems to have been the case. Enter: Columbus, whose story we know, who discovered the New World (after the Vikings and Chinese, but he got the credit).

Smoking was once thought not only harmless, but helpful in weight loss, as I mentioned, among other things.

And during the late 1800s, the US Patent Office was almost closed, since it was thought that anything worth discovering had already been discovered. Honest! Look it up!

We talked already about tomatoes. They were thought to be poison, or at least that's what most people—including the experts on the subjects—thought.

Ever hear of bloodletting and leeching to drain your blood? At the time, the then contemporary version of experts generally agreed that you could prevent or cure diseases, including high blood pressure, by draining blood out of the body. This killed a lot of people, including poet Lord Byron.

This practice wasn't abandoned until the late 1800s, past the era of the so-called "Enlightenment." Can you imagine a doctor sticking a leech on your arm to pull out blood to help you get over some disease? They really used to, and not all that long ago—within my grandfather's lifetime!

Remember the bubonic plague? Many cats were slaughtered during the period that it ravaged Europe in the 1300s since many people thought—starting with the Catholic Church and Pope Gregory IX (the experts of the time) in 1232—that they were agents of the devil, and the very thing that could have served to prevent the spread of plague was eradicated.

You could write a whole book on the subject of experts being wrong, and I suspect someone probably has.

I've included enough examples to make my point, and ignorance and superstition certainly aren't confined solely to years gone by. Certainly people in the past saw themselves as rational and enlightened, as we do now. We have the same ignorance and superstition today, it's just not called that. And it never occurs to most of us that we live in a world filled with it. Literally.

These were—and to a few, still are—incontestable, unquestioned truths. And humanity paid, and still pays, huge prices for the ignorance and superstition that fills our lives. We think we're so enlightened that we live in a world free of such superstition and ignorance, that we can't see the error of our own ways right now, and this totally blinds us to what really is happening (and sadly, this is also perpetuated by people in business and government who have an interest in maintaining our illusions and the status quo).

Getting back to where we started, please at least consider that simply because someone has a couple of letters after his or her name—or because they express an opinion—that they know what they are talking about in all matters about weight and nutrition. Perhaps they do, perhaps not. You have to do some studying and come to your own conclusions; it's your body, your health and your life that are at stake.

Certainly medical doctors are experts in certain arenas, but sadly, nutrition is generally not one of them.

Did you know that most medical schools require only a semester of a course on nutrition? And many med schools don't have even have this requirement!

Then there is another problem: experts disagree. One says x, the other says y. One seemingly legitimate peer reviewed study says one thing while another seemingly legitimate one says the total opposite. One says carbs are great while another one says they are not. And so on and so on, ad infinitum.

There are a couple of clues to look for, then you really need to trust your own personal common sense and judgment. First clue: where is the money? When a study commissioned by a tobacco company concludes that smoking isn't really a health hazard, do you believe them? When a study commissioned by the food industry concludes that processed foods, or eggs, meat, and so on, are healthy, do you believe them? The answer is hopefully no.

Now, here is the kicker. The USDA. They are the creators of the famous food pyramid, and supposedly the watchdogs of our health, but is composed largely of people who cycle in and out of the food industry. So when they say something, do we believe them? Sadly, the answer is often yes. No, of course they aren't always wrong, but this is where you really have to do some studying and use your common sense, or you will fall subject to the propaganda machine like most people have.

First of all, if you study the history of the food pyramid, based supposedly on objective science, but in fact, reflecting many other influences, political, business, and medical—plus a fair amount of ignorance on the subject of nutrition—the pyramid has constantly morphed. From butter having its own group, to recommending two servings of meat per day, to cutting back on meat and saturated fat. Hardly objective science, would you say? So why is today's food pyramid any less subjective and subject to error than the ones from the past?

Further, it's hard to believe that people from the industries who are selling things to eat, while on leave serving on the USDA, have our best interests at heart when putting these food pyramids together. It's science-based to a degree, but to a large extent politics plays a big role (watch <u>Plant Pure Nation</u>, referenced in the Resources chapter, to see what influences the food industry brings to bear on the lawmaking process).

Fifty or a hundred years from now, people will hopefully look at histories of what we now eat and shake their heads, wondering what the hell we were thinking eating chicken nuggets, a half pound of meat at one sitting, and drinking milk from a species not our own, and as adults at that. And hopefully the Standard American Diet will by then be relegated to the dustbin of history, along with killing cats, leeches, smoking, poisonous tomatoes, the flat earth concept, and all the rest.

Of course, I am not telling you to disregard what professionals in health, or any other field for that matter, are saying. All I am saying is to question whether what they tell you is true. They are fallible, as we all are, they are subject to fallacies and illusions as we all are, and can make mistakes just as easily.

Nowhere is this more evident than in the world of diet and eating. We are convinced that the contemporary diet of whatever the majority of Americans eat is the best of all possible worlds. Despite the fact that two thirds of us are overweight or obese. Despite the fact that we are raising overweight and obese children, who are more apt to become that same way as adults. Despite the fact that heart disease, diabetes, high blood pressure, all diseases that can be stopped and reversed through lifestyle changes, are rampant. Despite the fact that we have the highest health care costs in the world, it's what we know that just isn't so.

All of this points to how death from a heart attack, the leading cause of death in this country, is just as American as apple pie and hamburgers.

As Dr. John McDougall once observed, "People love to hear good things about their bad habits."

So when it comes to the opinion of your chosen expert, question it!

Here's another fallacy that people keep falling for: that the fad diet of the day will help them to lose and keep off weight, that diets are effective for both weight loss and weight maintenance and that the latest diet to come down the pike will somehow be more effective than all the others that never worked. That if they buy the newest book on Amazon, this will magically cure their problem. This is mostly wishful thinking, rather than a diet fallacy! Another one that's partly true, mostly not. We've touched on this a bit, but here's more.

People always want to believe in the next miracle cure that comes along. Sure, you can lose weight with a fad diet. People do it all the time. You can lose weight by cutting off your arm, too. You can lose weight by literally starving yourself, by eating absolutely nothing or by going on a hunger strike. Not too smart. Any of them.

Remember what I talked about earlier, that weight isn't the problem but that weight is the symptom of the problem? Well, the fad diet, like any of these diets we're discussing, addresses the symptom. It's giving lozenges to smokers to stop the coughing. It's giving driving lessons to drunks that get into accidents. It's building sea walls around coastal cities as a solution to the rising sea level.

And of course we all know what happens to us at the end of a fad diet or if we've paid a bunch of money for liposuction by a doctor who should have known better, gone to a fat farm for thousands of dollars, or some such thing—where we've lost 50 pounds in some impossibly short period of time. The very notion of "diet" implies "end of diet" or to stop dieting.

Not only have we not established healthy eating habits to replace our bad habits, we REWARD ourselves for being so virtuous as to have lost 50 pounds. What the hell do we think is going to happen? Are we going back to eating like we once did, somehow magically gaining the control we never had?

Nonsense. We may lose 10-50-100 pounds, but unless we've adopted a new way of eating, i.e changed our eating totally, the only thing that will eventually happen is that our old habits will reassert themselves, and we will start eating the way we used to eat again with the same consequences: physical, mental and emotional.

Not only is this futile, but it's even unhealthier than having not done it at all. My guess is that you can verify this from your own experience, right or wrong?

As I mentioned, only 5% of people who go on a diet and lose weight actually keep it off for an extended period of time. According to ABC news, Americans try to lose weight on average 4 to 5 times per year (the story didn't say how many were successful), so you do the math. The statistics are abysmal. Which is to say, if you take the old route, the diet route, your odds are equally abysmal. Virtually zero.

5. "Where Do You Get Your Protein?" (Be ready for this one!)

If someone is foolish enough to mention to anyone that they stay away from meat, fish, and dairy (See the chapter: "Silence is Golden"), invariably they will get a question like the above. It will usually be a sincere question, but said in the wrong tone, it often comes off as challenging.

And without fail, the person doing the questioning isn't someone who avoids meat, dairy or fish. It's a typical response of a person who (a) hasn't studied the science on this or most areas regarding nutrition but who thinks he or she is qualified to speak about it, and (b), feels threatened by a person who is avoiding things they know good and well aren't healthy.

But consider: if someone ever says they love meat, do they ever get asked where they get their fiber? Their micronutrients? Their antioxidants?

Have they ever met anyone who was sickened—or hospitalized—because of protein deficiency? If you eat a varied, plant based diet, it doesn't happen so long as you're getting enough calories, and not getting all the calories you do get through junk vegan food. Period.

But unless you have been living on a desert island or under a rock, you no doubt know people who have been sickened, hospitalized, or died from heart disease, a stroke, type II diabetes, diverticulitis, kidney failure, breast, prostate, or colon cancer, and so on. All these are primarily lifestyle diseases. Diseases we quite literally choose to have or to increase our odds of contracting--whether we want to look at it this way or not--which are largely caused and promoted by eating meat, eggs, dairy, fish and added oils and fats.

Diseases which could be for the most part totally avoided—and in some cases actually reversed—by switching to a whole foods plant based way of eating.

But we sometimes hear the objection that plant proteins aren't a complete protein. This fallacy, which is still with us, was started in the 1970's in a book called *Diet For a Small Planet*, where the author stated that it was necessary to combine plant proteins to get a healthful balance.

And later, after science had proved this not to be the case, and the author of the book (Francis Lappè) had disavowed her original thesis, the damage had been done. So here we are nearly fifty years later with many people still believing this.

We also hear people doubting that you get enough strength or energy from plant proteins. Ever hear of Shaolin monks? They really exist, not just in kung fu movies. Most of them eat a totally whole foods plant based diet and they get enough protein, on their veggie-based diet, to be capable of incredible physical feats.

Remember Mike Tyson, former heavyweight champion of the world? He's now a vegan. Yup! Ask him how HE gets HIS protein!

And even Arnold Schwarzenegger has looked into and advocates starting to move in the direction of vegan eating. In an article from Breitbart.com, he was asked how prospective bodybuilders are supposed to build muscle without meat, and he replied, "I have seen many bodybuilders and weight lifters that are vegetarians. You can get your protein source many different ways."

There are countless examples of other athletes who are plant fueled as well. They run ultra marathons, win Ultimate Fighting championships, and so on, all powered by plants. Are you going to accuse Shaolin monks, Arnold, Mike Tyson, and various UFC champions of wimpdom because they don't eat meat or of not getting enough protein? I didn't think so!

I will take my chances with my supposedly protein deficient diet, thank you very much. If you do the research as I have done, you will no doubt come to this conclusion as well.

6. Diet Fallacies, Conclusion

Well, here you have gotten a bunch of the larger diet fallacies and there are many, many more. Part of the process of losing weight and keeping it off is educating yourself as to why you have the problem in the first place, and focusing on lifestyle change, rather than weight loss. ***You have to lose the diet mentality***. Because, without that, you will repeat the same mistakes.

I hope this has been encouraging, in the sense of showing you why you've had difficulties in the past, and honest in that I'm telling you what you NEED to hear, and not what you WANT to hear. Yes, I'm like you. If there was a way I could eat junk foods moderately, I'd be all for it. If I could learn to drink moderately, I'd be all for it, but that isn't going to happen, and I hope you don't have to go through what I've had to with food, booze, drugs (which I didn't mention, but which is a part of my story as well), and cigarettes, to find that out the hard way, and many times over.

You CAN get off the diet merry go round for good, it is totally possible, and you CAN get your eating under control. And when you get your eating under control by feeding the body the foods it needs, your weight will go down. You will have addressed the CAUSE of the problem, and created a different effect.

Normal eating = normal weight.

7. A New Direction
(a.k.a., Now What?)

So how, in this abnormal world, do we begin to start eating normally? The first step, as I've discussed a bit, is to discover the nature of the problem, which is what we've been doing. The next step is to explore this new direction, after convincing ourselves of its necessity, or at least having become open to the possibility.

The native diets in other parts of the world that keep people with a weight more considered "normal," and where people live the longest use a different formula. A traditionally developed formula that is whole foods, plant based, the basis of this entire way of eating that I am advocating. And they typically don't diet. Why not? THEY DON'T HAVE TO!

Fortunately for us we can create and have our own version of the same thing wherever we happen to be. It's delicious, healthy, and will allow the body to return to, and maintain, a sensible, realistic weight for itself. It will probably increase our life expectancies as well.

We are not limited by geography and small numbers of available regional foods, such as the corn, beans, squash and maize of Mexico, another traditional diet that maintained both weight and health, until recently. We have foods from the entire world at our disposal, and they can be terrific!

Again, please don't spend a lot of time thinking that this eating plan will enable you to get into a size seven dress. Maybe it will, maybe not. If you or someone else wants to become a sex object, knock yourself out, but that's not what this book is about. It's about helping you to get to a sane, healthy weight that is right for your particular body and body type, not about recreating you into someone else's fantasy about what the ideal body type is. And that's doomed to fail at the outset because the goal is unrealistic.

Isn't it time for us to get it through our heads that diets don't work, and to consider this new direction?

A new direction is just that. New. It will be something out of your current field of vision, and probably out of your comfort zone as well. The whole idea of a "whole foods plant based" diet may be just that. But it will work. It worked, and is still working, for many, many people, and it will work for you. How badly do you want to get your eating under control? Are you willing to do what it takes to lose that weight and keep it off?

Or are you going to continue to be seduced by the siren cry of "mañana?" Or, "I know it's a healthier way to live, but now is not the time because ...It's busy at work....When the kids have left home..., When the holidays are over"...(fill in the blank)? You will find plenty of time for a trip to the ER or to dialysis, I am sure.

Or will you be one of those who disagrees, puts this book down, and then goes to find the latest diet to hit number one on the best seller charts, that will deliver the same, law-conformable results that diets have always gotten them in the past?

Do you think that a person sitting alone in their home, as an older adult, grossly overweight, with only their cat, a quart of ice cream and their TV to keep them company, is going to regret the food choices they've made in their lives, especially if they now know what you know?

Do you think a person in that same situation, having lost their eyesight and a foot to diabetes is going to be saying, "All that rich food was worth every bite!?"

I realize you are now in an awkward position. You are beginning to understand how and why the old ways of dieting don't work, and never will work, despite the ads and despite your desperate yearning for them to deliver what they promise. But the new way is new. Perhaps unappealing as well. All sorts of objections may be coming up for you. I am not asking for your agreement, but what I am asking for is your willingness to become willing, and your willingness to try to take in some new ideas. For without at least that, nothing can or will change for you.

I realize and understand all these objections you are having about a new way of eating—everyone needs to deal with them, if they are to move forward, and I did as well. Change means change. Dealing with these objections will be a part of another book, to be released in the future, if it isn't out already. All you have to bring is your willingness to learn.

It pays to be ahead of the rest of the herd on things about your own health, believe me! Despite what others may say and how they might try to influence you.

Fortunately, more and more people have found the connection between weight, diet, and health. And you can lead like these people, or you can follow the herd, if you are still around and are able to walk. If someone looks ahead a few years, and if he keeps eating as he now does, do you think, when his cardiologist tells him that he has only a few months to live, that his thought will be "All those steaks and fries were totally worth it?"

But you can make these changes for yourself right now. You do not need society, your friends, or your family to approve or disapprove of your desire for your own good health or your proper weight. For there ALWAYS will be people who disapprove and who try to discourage, thinking they know better. The direction I'm suggesting works wonders, but only if you are willing to resist the naysayers, both the ones outside yourself and the ones inside yourself, that speak in the same way.

8. Just Say Yes
(Well, to the right things!)

There was a book called *The Yes Man* (written by Danny Wallace, not to be confused with a movie starring Jim Carey with the same title) written a number of years ago about an English guy, who seemed to have everything going for him. He had a great job; he was a journalist in London. He had a flat, friends, and stature in the community. In short, he had everything on the outside that seemed exactly what a young man would want, except that his girlfriend had broken up with him. He was miserable, unhappy, lonely, saw no purpose or meaning in his life, and had no idea what to do about it.

One day on a bus, he happened to be sitting next to an Indian gentleman, and they got into a discussion. The Indian gentleman said to him, "You know your problem? You say no. All the time. You need to start saying YES."

The man had an epiphany. He realized in that moment that he was living a life of negation, saying no to every new opportunity that came by, and in short, keeping his life exactly the way it was, maintaining the status quo, because of negation.

He resolved in that moment to spend the next year saying yes. He sought every opportunity to say yes. He left no "yes" unsaid. He said "yes" to the most unlikely of opportunities.

And in short, his life totally changed and totally transformed. And he got married!

I am not suggesting that you say "yes" to every opportunity to send money to some scam in Nigeria, or to get a free estimate for your siding for your house, nor do I think this is the point of the book—but think about this: every time we say "no", it is the voice of the status quo talking. It is the voice of business as usual.

"Every time that we say 'no', we maintain the status quo."

Now, I am also not suggesting that every word in this book you are now reading has the force, impact, or veracity of the voice of God, written on tablets brought down from Sinai, but I am suggesting that as you find yourself resisting the new ideas in this book, instead of rejecting them out of hand, consider them. Find a way at least in a small part of yourself to say "Yes." Remember the results the Yes Man got.

Feel free to do your own research. The ideas in this book are scientifically verified. I didn't pull them out of the air. They will help you lose weight, and they will get you on the back on the path to a normal weight and vibrant health. Isn't this what you want?

Let's get something clear at the outset: weight and weight loss are primarily controlled by the number of calories we put into our bodies, above or below our daily needs. Period. Exercise is a factor, but it's mostly controlled by our eating. Yes, I know there is lots, lots more that goes into it, but I am simplifying to make a point, and the basic point is quite accurate.

Our problem is that, as we are now, we eat foods that are tasty, nutritionally deficient and high in calories. We need to change that to eating foods that are tasty, nutritionally loaded, and low in calories. And THIS is the new direction. And THAT will take off the weight.

By the way, that last paragraph is my entire program in a nutshell—if you can hear and implement that, you will not only lose weight, but keep it off for good.

9. The Emotional Side of the Coin (Or, You can't think your way out of this)

Here is a new idea for you: you will never lose weight if you try to do it by strict logic. Your logical mind simply does not have the strength or speed to be the only force in helping you lose weight. It is very tough, if not impossible, to break or change habits strictly by logic. A logical mind can only go so far, but it needs the help of your emotions, which are much faster and stronger.

You don't need me to tell you why you need to do something about your eating. You have been telling yourself this for years. You know about the consequences, and it's gotten you to exactly where you are right now. This is your logical mind at work. The logical mind is great for some things, like balancing a checkbook, memorizing things, or using Excel, but as a motivational force, it doesn't work well. It's the wrong tool for the job. And that is not its job. You tell me, has it worked so far?

Let's see if we can find a way to also address the problem emotionally. If you haven't done so already, let's start by writing out a list of what you want to get by losing the weight that you want to lose.

Is it vibrant health you want? Is it more energy? Is it feeling better about yourself? Stop. Literally, before you read any further, put the book down, take out a piece of paper or start a Word document, spend 10 or 15 minutes without censorship writing out every imaginable good thing that can and will come when you get your eating under control and your weight regains some normalcy. Ignore the voices that say "That will never happen," or "Hah!" or whatever version of negation happens to be the one that is yours, and that comes to the fore when you do this exercise. Or the voices that tell you that this exercise is silly and that don't want you to do it.

Write things that are real for YOU. Things that YOU want. For after all, even though your family, friends and co-workers will benefit by your getting your eating under control, it's really about you and what you can get for yourself. And you don't need to show this list to ANYONE!

How will you look physically? How will you feel physically? Emotionally? What opportunities will you have that are now closed to you? Let your imagination soar!

Write twenty-five things. And don't stop until you get to twenty-five, though there are at least that many, and more!

Then take out another piece of paper, or start another Word file and write what won't happen if you continue to let your eating be out of control. What you will lose? What opportunities you'll be foregoing? How you will feel when you look at yourself in the mirror? What about the relationships that will be damaged or will never happen? Let your mind wander and write another fifty things.

I'm including some things to help you get started in the process, but you can fill in a whole lot more that are personal to you:

- Your weight will come off. The weight comes off by itself, not as a goal, but as a byproduct of eating differently and healthier. Remember, your body wants to heal.

- You'll have better health. Probably fewer colds and other illnesses, among other things.

- You'll have more energy.

- You'll feel better about yourself.

- You'll have less self-judgment.

- You will look better to yourself and others.

- You'll be able to stop beating yourself up about your eating.

- You'll stop obsessing about food.

- You'll have fewer food cravings, and at some point be totally free from them.

- You'll save lots of time (I'll explain this in another place).

- You'll have higher self-esteem.

- You'll have a better sex life. Or you'll start <u>having</u> a sex life!

- You will sleep better.

- You'll reduce danger of hypertension, high cholesterol, heart disease, diabetes, cancer, strokes, and so on.

- You'll very possibly save money on doctor bills.

- You definitely won't be spending money on junk foods.

- The odds are you will live longer since you will be lowering your chances of getting many diseases.

- This will be the end of yo-yo dieting.

- You will very possibly experience less depression.

- You'll be motivated to help your kids eat healthier foods.

- You'll have FAR less beating yourself up—at least as far as food is concerned.

- You'll have a feeling of being in control of your food and your life.

- You will look younger.

- You will have more chances for promotions at work.

- You will have a success you will be proud to share with your friends, if they ask (but don't tell anyone right away what you are doing—we'll talk of this later).

Put both these lists somewhere you can see them every day, but make sure it's a private place. This is your business and not anyone else's. In fact, it's better if you see it <u>more</u> than once every day. Rather than looking at everything each time you view this list, though, take a look at only one or two of the items at a time. Let them become real for you as you glance at them. Look at different things each day. Take some time and let yourself get emotional about them. Close your eyes and let your imagination go where it may. Let yourself experience the pain of not having the good things about controlling your eating in your life. Just one or two, that's all we can handle in the moment.

And conversely, imagine yourself having these things in your life. Imagine how your life will be changed and transformed when you have these things. Let these emotions act in conjunction with your intellect to help push you forward to adopting and embracing this new eating plan. Focus on different things on your lists every day, so this exercise is new and fresh each day, otherwise it will become rote and lose its effectiveness. This will help you both get and keep the emotional "oomph" you need to bring this new way of eating into your life.

Remember, if anyone thinks that their high fat, animal protein centered diet, with minimal fiber, is going to get them anything but a one-way ticket to obesity, increasingly bad health, and ultimately their own premature demise, they had better look at the facts. If anybody thinks that giving this stuff up long enough to lose weight and then to start back eating the same crap again is going to change anything at all in the long run, they need to wake up.

They are on a collision course with reality, and reality always wins.

I know a change as I am suggesting is going into new areas for you, into uncharted territory, but without the aid of the emotions combined with the intellect, you will turn around and go back to business as usual. Your "no" will reassert itself. Your "but" will reassert itself. And believe me, your butt will as well!

Let's become yes men and women! And if you really want to stretch yourself, you can extend this exercise to other opportunities as well. Say hello to strangers! Realize they are friends you haven't met yet. Smile at people you don't know! Most of them aren't axe murderers, you know! Let someone go ahead of you in traffic! Instead of disagreeing with someone, ask, "Is there anything in what this person is saying?" or "How can I take in something I disagree with in a new way?"

Remember, you can be right, or you can regain your normal, lower, healthy and proper weight. Your choice. You can have "business as usual," for the rest of your life or you can begin to make a change in your thinking. Regaining your normal weight simply won't happen if you keep the same thinking and attitudes. Be willing to be wrong!

10. The Bad News
(Yep, there's always bad news)

And as true as all this is, there is a lighter side to successful weight loss through whole foods plant based eating as well.

After you drop weight, you will have to go clothes shopping.

You will have to get used to a new sense of yourself.

You will constantly have to field questions about "how did you lose all that weight?"

Weight loss won't solve all the problems in your life. No matter how heavy or light you are, you will still be you, with all your habits and inclinations, good and bad. And you will still have to pay the rent or the mortgage, taxes, and so on.

But you know what? It will solve a lot of your problems, and often the ones you do have will seem far less important or significant.

And you may well realize that what you called "emotional eating" was more a result of addictive eating and the emotions that ensued from that than any emotional difficulties.

Hopefully nobody tries to hide behind "I'm an emotional eater." That's often just another way of saying, "It's not my fault" and "I'm a hapless victim of circumstance," and blaming something other than themselves and their decisions and choices for their difficulties. I know this isn't true for everyone, but allow the possibility that it may be true for you.

Plus, unhealthy foods have a way of stirring less than positive emotions up in us. We get locked into inner places of self-pity, self-hatred, self-deprecation and so on, brought about and stirred up by the poisons we are putting down our throats. We then claim "emotional eating," but please don't buy this argument! Stop poisoning yourself with crap foods, and those emotions will begin to heal, and shift. Besides, if you <u>really</u> want to become an emotional eater, learn to love this new way of eating!

However, the really bad news...and this is the most difficult part of all...if you are ready...is that you will have to do things differently. If you want the weight to stay off, you will need to take the actions that make this happen. Your thinking about food will need to change, as we've discussed. Your feelings about food will have to change and, as I said, your behavior will need to change.

And it isn't that difficult, it's just different. We were not born overeaters. We didn't beat ourselves up mercilessly when we were very little for drinking too much out of our bottles or mothers' breasts. This overeating as adults is all learned behavior. As is the self-deprecation. Part of the problem is that we are all creatures of habit. This is what has gotten us to where we are now, and this is what has to change.

We need to replace unhelpful, injurious, and unhealthy habits with ones that are conducive to health, happiness and a long life, and there is the whole arena of food addiction that adds another layer to this.

11. Addictive Eating, (Or, "Me? A Junkie?")

The first couple of bites may be really good. The silkiness of the chocolate, the crunch of the nuts, the little land mines of sweet crunchiness built in around them—and then the craving starts in force. Where logic would tell us to stop eating after a half a cup of ice cream, it is generally and invisibly superseded by an insatiable urge to keep putting the stuff into our mouths until the half pint, or the pint, is either gone or we are so sick we can't keep eating.

This same scenario could be repeated, just substituting your favorite junk food, be it potato chips, Oreos, French fries, pizza, Wing Dings, or whatever. Modify a few adjectives, and the same event repeats almost indefinitely

(On a personal note, how many full bags of olive oil potato chips have I personally gone through this with? No idea, but far TOO many!)

A thought of a food item occurs, we see it in the grocery store, or somehow the notion of "food" gets into our mind. Perhaps we see an ad, a TV show, or a twinge of real hunger engenders the notion. Even if there is a momentary resistance, action follows the cravings and the impulse to eat. Upon the first bite, the cravings kick in, the control goes out the window, and the inevitable consequence occurs: out of control eating. It starts the same way, it ends the same way. Deja vu all over again.

We attribute this to personal weakness and that we have no will power. Have you not yet realized, like we discussed, that junk foods are engineered to make them irresistible? Quite literally created in such a way that once you start eating them, you are physically unable to stop?

Now the good news: you are not some weak-willed, spineless person. You very well may not have an eating disorder (remember, though, I am not a health care professional). You are also not some sort of horrible person because you eat like this. You have become hooked, without your knowledge or consent, on foods manufactured to be hyperirresistable. Uberirresistable

You are suffering, as Dr. David Kessler, author of *The End of Overeating* (see Resources chapter) calls it, from "conditioned hypereating." One bite of certain foods, and you can't stop. Certain other foods are little or no problem. Ever hear of someone who couldn't stop eating bananas? (Monkeys excluded, of course). Quinoa? Broccoli? No, of course not. They are healthy foods, which generally don't become addictive.

So let's look at food through the lens of addiction, instead of calling it "conditioned hypereating." It's somewhat similar to drugs and alcohol, except the process of developing a food addiction doesn't have to take anywhere near as long. Food scientists engineer this stuff to be instantly addictive. Don't believe me? Look at your record.

These titillating junk foods have as a part of their structure, as you now know, sugar, fat and salt, plus artificial flavors added to create this craving. Remove this stuff from the foods and what do you have? Cardboard. Flavorless flakes. Stuff you would never consider eating.

Processed and junk foods began to be heavily marketed in the 1980s, and, to no surprise, that's when the American waistline began to expand as well. Their allure comes not just from their convenience, but largely from these various combinations of sugar, salt, and fat. They are designed for maximum appeal, taste and texture. Of course! Why not? Why shouldn't the manufacturers make the stuff taste good? That's the producers' job, to sell food! This isn't some evil conspiracy to make us fat, it's American capitalism at work, out to make a buck. Sadly, though, it's created a nation of food junkies. Specifically, junk food junkies.

The other part of their job, although they don't say this to the general public, and perhaps would be offended to hear me saying this, is to create addictive behavior through creating foods that you will be incapable of stopping eating once you start.

Not only did the food industry start catering to our desires for ease, convenience, and comfort, but the food manufacturers started selling us foods that were highly palatable, highly addictive and highly unhealthy. They are calorically dense and nutrient deficient, plus we are powerless against overeating this stuff because of their composition.

No, one packaged dinner isn't going to kill us (that is, if we can stop with one). But what is the effect of eating these things daily? What if we eat them habitually? What about fast foods and binge-inducing foods becoming a big part of our steady diet? What if these foods that have fiber removed and are low in nutrients with chemical additives become what our "normal" is? What if all of our own personal food choices are made by corporations?

We know the answer when we look in the mirror in the morning. We are consuming more calories. We find we are powerless to stop eating this stuff. The corporations don't give a damn about you or me. They are profit driven, in case you haven't noticed.

And if you continue down their primrose path, you will see your same oversized reflection in the mirror for the rest of your life, only bigger, and bigger!

As we discussed, there is no solution taking the usual routes. The path of dieting. The path everyone else takes. What do we do when we go on a diet? We deprive ourselves of all or most of these foods. We feel deprived. Diets are never additive; they make our lives smaller and more restricted. We put our bodies –and our minds--into starvation mode.

And yes, the pounds will come off, often with great difficulty, and what happens at the end, after we've lost ten, twenty or a hundred pounds? We reward ourselves. With just one bite, or just one bowl of ice cream, or some such. Then a few days later, another, then the next day another, and quickly, before we know it, we're off to the races again, gaining weight as if the reduction had never happened. Sound familiar?

Remember the quote "Those who cannot remember the past are doomed to repeat it" by George Santayana? This doesn't apply just to all those other people, this applies to us. Right here. Right now.

So let's talk about how this addiction rears its ugly head in uncontrolled eating and food cravings. We know what we can't stop eating: processed foods, restaurant foods, colas and soft drinks, and certain home cooked foods with sugar, salt and fat as major parts of the ingredients list.

How many servings are there in a quart of ice cream? In a bag of chips, or a bag of cookies, despite what it says on the label we try not to read? ONE! We lie to ourselves that we will have just a bowl, or a few chips or cookies, then we catch ourselves thinking that a few more won't hurt, then we find ourselves eating more and more, getting more and more uncomfortable, then when there's only a bit more, we say "since there's only a bit more..." and then we kill the package or container of food we started.

We feel like hell physically and we beat ourselves up emotionally for being weak-willed, and so on, only to repeat the same cycle again, telling ourselves "well, I'll just have a bite or two." This is the result of the food industry at work, creating addictive behavior, with all its concomitant lying to ourselves.

This behavior isn't limited to cookies and ice cream. It could be pizza, steak, ribs, pancakes, all you can eat restaurants, buckets of fried chicken, or anything food that's harmful and addictive. Does this sound familiar? We invariably find ourselves in the position of being unable to stop eating. The combinations of sugar, salt and fat in the foods we buy have created an irresistible craving.

There is natural hunger and there is a craving. Natural hunger can be satisfied. A craving cannot. Do you know the difference? If you have ever been on a 24-hour fast, you will get a sense of what natural hunger really is. Alternatively, you could eat a light dinner and then skip breakfast as an experiment. You will probably experience true hunger. (By the way, skipping breakfast is a recipe for overeating later in the day, so it's not a good idea.)

Isn't the impossibility of satisfaction always an element in any yielding to the cravings of an addiction? Is there anything real in the titillation of junk food or does it promise a satisfaction, but which winds up delivering only a momentary, high-priced burst of pleasure? Are we really thinking that we will ever be able to eat enough? As we take that first bite of a chip or slice of pizza do we ever consider we won't stop without having totally pigged out, or at the very least having overeaten past where we planned to?

Looked at through a clear lens, as we discussed, continuing addictive eating is a recipe for hopelessness and despair.

Eat junk now, pay later.

Sadly, food addiction is *just* as real as drug, alcohol and cigarette addiction, despite the dispute within the health care community about this and despite that people don't wake up in the gutter with cookie crumbs on their faces. The big difference, at least as far as I can see, is that the withdrawal isn't anywhere near as severe. However, the consequences of the addiction are just as deadly and debilitating, and we even EXPECT these consequences as we get older in the form of disease of lifestyle. So it really doesn't matter what you call it: addiction, habit, addiction-like, or whatever. It still is going to do you in, unless you find a way to change it.

The problem is that it is largely invisible (again, that word), not discussed, and in fact it is even subsidized by the government through their farm subsidy programs (which means the government is also subsidizing the health care crisis, by the way). In order to combat food addiction in yourself, you have to go against a lot of current thinking and behavior—the behavior of the ⅔ of the people who are overweight or obese.

What are some of the other characteristics of an addiction? One is that when you stop feeding the addiction, whether drugs, alcohol, cigarettes or food, you will feel this craving for the stuff you aren't putting into your system. The problem is that addictive cravings are insatiable. As you have learned, there is no such thing as enough. You've perhaps heard, regarding alcohol, that "one's too many, and a thousand's not enough." Food addiction is the same. One bite of an addictive food, and you are generally off and running, and who knows when you will stop.

We can look at food cravings as "Addiction Withdrawal Light." Not as severe as the DT's of alcohol withdrawal, but real nonetheless. Note, though, this doesn't make them any less pernicious or less real.

Of course, your inner Evil Twin, your lying inner Mr. or Ms. Hyde, can and generally will come in at this point, and, after convincing you to take "just one bite," say something like, "Well, I got away with just one bite, so obviously I don't have a problem. I'll take another." Maybe you will actually stop with the one bite, though this thought will occur again in a day or two, maybe even a week later, with very predictable consequences. You're pigging out again very shortly.

You change behavior by changing behavior, not by trying to cheat or pretending that the problem has gone away or that you have overcome the addiction. You cannot overcome your addiction. It's impossible. You will have it for life. But, and this is critical, you can control it by abstinence. To keep the wild animal in its cage, you need to lock the door and throw away the key. Through abstinence.

Someone may not choose to call this sort of eating an addiction. Fine. I am certain they will agree with me, though, that with the foods we are talking about, once we start eating, we tend not to stop. This designation I am making calling this an addiction is about helping people see the truth of a situation, no matter what they may choose to call it. And frankly, it's immaterial whether it falls into anyone's definition of "addiction."

Your Evil Twin, the lying voice of temptation, is NOT your friend! The ET deals in enticing, half-truths. Remember, Mr. Hyde ultimately destroyed Dr. Jekyll. He doesn't have to destroy you!

The bottom line on the lie of trying "just one bite" is, it doesn't work. Do that, and it's downhill from there. Whether immediately or later.

And you *will* have food cravings. They are part of the process. The process of losing the weight you want to lose. Remember when you have them, it's your clue that you are getting slimmer, healthier, more attractive, sexier, more confident, more responsible for your life. The list goes on and on.

So look at this way: cravings are a good thing...

And by resisting temptation, you become stronger.

Another temptation will be in the form of your ET telling you "I'm starving." Nonsense. You may be hungry, but please don't tell yourself you are starving. That's total BS. If you are emaciated, sitting in the dirt somewhere in Africa with flies in your eyes that you don't have the strength to chase away, then yes, you are starving. But not as you are. This is the voice of the Evil Twin, and if you indulge in hanging on to these thoughts, in dwelling on them, on tormenting yourself with them, you will pay.

In the same way, when the ET tells you that you are being deprived, it's essential to remember that this new way of eating really is additive, not depriving. These feelings are a part of the process of addiction withdrawal. You can get negative. You can complain, go into self-pity, start cursing me (as you no doubt will) and all the other stuff that the ET will throw at you, but again, it's all part of the process. See the section on deprivation for more material.

Isn't it better, and smarter, to remind yourself of what you are *adding* by surfing these cravings, riding them out and allowing them to pass?

You will be adding benefit and value to your life. You are depriving yourself, if you are depriving yourself of anything at all, of being overweight, increasingly unhealthy, feeling unattractive, lowering your job and promotion prospects, of feeling less sexy, and so on. May we all be so deprived!

You are *adding* the other things we've mentioned, and the things from your own list as well and it's important to constantly remind yourself of that if you start thinking "I can't eat this stuff anymore." If you are in a literal jail that serves nothing but prison fare, that may be true, there will be things you "can't" eat. But you are probably not there, any more than you are starving in Africa. Of course you *can eat* unhealthy foods. But if you are smart, and throw your weight in the direction of the new, you may *choose* not to yield or succumb. We believe what we tell ourselves repeatedly. True or otherwise.

What we are seeking is the middle ground. On the one hand, we have the desire to eat, as opposed to cravings. On the other hand, we have the satisfaction of natural hunger through healthy eating. Certainly we have an instinctive need to eat, which must be dealt with, but it doesn't have to be the burden that it now is. We need to begin to distinguish the real, and rather quiet voice, of true hunger as it calls us not just to eat, but to nourish ourselves.

12. Food Cravings, (Or, "Betcha can't eat just one!")

You've heard these stories about soldiers and journalists who come back from war zones, from seeing all sorts of horrible things, from being in constant mortal danger. Guess what? These people often return to these places because their lives are no longer as stimulating. They return to rape, pillaging, destruction, plunder, and mortal danger because they're craving a stimulation they aren't getting.

Our taste buds are exactly the same way with food. We hyper-stimulate them with totally deadly, unhealthy quantities of sugar, salt and fat, repeatedly, and surprise, we want more!

We live in a world of hyper-stimulation, of food porn. The food we eat today, the processed and restaurant stuff, just like pornography, is titillating but ultimately not satisfying. What is titillation? It's a like a tickling, a sort of inveigling temptation that lures, allures, and never satisfies, but which we continue to want to feed, as it were.

Have you begun to see that there is nothing real in the titillation of junk and processed foods? It promises what it can't deliver.

The word titillation means: "to excite or arouse agreeably," often with sexual overtones. The media is this way, with all its pseudo sexuality. The attraction of the appearances of movie stars, and the superficiality of it, that we all decry, are but are drawn to nonetheless.

The line between craving, a titillating experience, and natural hunger is often blurred in our minds. It's pretty apparent with experience, but we often confuse them. Since we're usually in the middle of a craving of some sort, we don't recognize natural hunger when we experience it.

And, isn't there always the element of the impossibility of satisfaction in any yielding to the cravings of an addiction? Is there anything real in the titillation of junk food, or sexual titillation, or is it empty promises of satisfaction that just don't deliver? Real hunger can be satisfied. The false hunger of a craving, of food titillation, cannot be.

Titillation of all kinds ultimately leads us to the point of despair where we see, perhaps later in life when it may be too late, that which we imagine sexually can and never come to be. Social situations can never be improved by being drunk, or relaxation can never be achieved by self-stimulation through addictive smoking. It eventually leads us to see also that the food we can't stop eating, that makes us fat, sick, and lethargic, can never ultimately be satisfying. Do you see yourself in any of this?

Wouldn't it make sense to address this NOW, instead of later, when it's too late to do anything about it?

Looked at through the lens of what the future may offer, titillation is a sure-fire recipe for hopelessness and despair, no matter what form it takes.

Craving is a combination of an intense physical desire, and a psychological obsession. You think constantly about food. You salivate at the thought; the tempting, repeating, alluring constant thought. Not the same thing as hunger, by a long shot. Except in cases of literal starvation, no one has obsessions about brown rice or asparagus.

Our taste buds have been seduced by the sugar, salt, and fat into thinking, or at least into accepting, that the crap we are eating is what we really want. Well, it certainly is what the addictive craving for the trigger ingredients wants, but as we have seen elsewhere, the body doesn't really want or need this stuff at all; the craving is the addiction talking, and the body will get diseased and obese when we eat too much of whatever we are craving. Does the physical craving for tobacco or alcohol or cocaine mean that this is what the body wants or needs or is normal for it? No, of course not.

I know of only two ways to get rid of food cravings. First, is by not feeding them. You feed them directly by eating foods they want, by pretending that it's going to be "just one," or by going on some foolish maintenance diet that says to have small portions of pizza or potato chips or ice cream, which invariably, sooner or later, leads to larger and larger portions.

You cannot put out a fire by pouring gasoline on it, particularly when the fuel is the high octane stuff of junk and processed foods you feed yourself. How can you possibly expect cravings to go away by giving yourself the very things that are causing them in the first place?

It's at this point that someone always points out they know someone whose eating was once out of control, and now are able to have just small amounts. Great. Perhaps they can. Good for them.

As we've discussed, you are not that person. You are unique. You are different and you are yourself, both for better and for worse. If you could have developed that control, you would have done so a long time ago. So please, don't waste your time entertaining such thoughts. Junk foods are junk foods, and whether or not you can control your consumption, they are still doing very bad things to your body. There are people who smoke until they are 90 and then die of something unrelated, but that's not an intelligent argument for smoking, either.

And this person who supposedly has food cravings under control? We see only their outer world. We do not see the inner struggles they no doubt have to contend with constantly to maintain this "control." For however long this so-called control lasts.

The first way to get rid of these cravings is to not feed them at all. We do this by eliminating the foods we've discussed so far: processed foods and foods that are heavy in sugar, salt, and fat. No matter where you are eating, focusing on whole foods, plant based eating will get rid of the cravings for foods that are high in calories and low in nutrients over time.

And if this concept seems a bit "out there" for you, if this seems like hippie crunchy granola flaky stuff, consider again that Kaiser Permanente Health (the nation's largest health insurer) recommends this way of eating, both for weight and for health. And so do many other health professionals as well—see the appendix.

By focusing on adding the highly nutritious, low calorie, whole food plant based foods, and eliminating the others, you will effectively starve the cravings, a bit at a time, out of existence.

The other way to get rid of food cravings is a part of the first. It's the passage of time. The longer you stay away from the addictive foods without eating any, the less frequently you will experience the cravings. And down the road, they may come rarely or never.

"But wait", you say, "what about the cravings I'm having NOW?!"

Good question. The first important thing to understand is that cravings are a symptom of the addiction, as we discussed, and are perfectly normal. It doesn't mean you are failing, that you are weak-willed, that you are doing something wrong, that you are doomed to go back to overeating.

There are a few ways to deal with them in the moment. First thing, when you are not in the middle of them, is to go back to your list of what you will gain by your healthy eating. Starting with your weight loss. What do you want from this? Why are you reading this book right now?

Second, embrace the cravings. Don't try to get rid of them. You can't. They will just pop up again, bigger and stronger. Acknowledge that yes, you want to eat! You still have the choice as to what you do, but lying about it, telling yourself "I don't want that French fry," simply never works. Yes, you want the damn thing!! No one knows what you will do in the moment, but by lying and saying "I don't want this," or "I can't," will effectively be setting yourself up to binge.

Acknowledging and accepting can win the day. Lying never will.

So let's look at what we get by yielding to a food craving. Nobody takes that first bite thinking in any real or serious way about obesity, heart disease, type II diabetes, increased cancer risk and all the rest. Nobody has ever been wheeled into the ER, on the way to get a quadruple bypass, thinking "I am so happy I succumbed to temptation every time!"

Of course, though, we may lie to ourselves and say, "just a bite," or "I'll get back on the wagon tomorrow," or the famous, "Screw it." And sure, the first bite or two tastes good, but then the craving kicks in. And do you know why you continue? To avoid the discomfort of not yielding to the temptation, and to avoid the temporary discomfort of not eating.

That's it. That's the payoff. Not my observation, but it's 100% accurate. Avoiding the temporary discomfort of not eating in that moment. We don't see ourselves in time, unfortunately, but only in the moment. What we choose to do in the moment has the potential to affect our entire lives, and nowhere is this more true than with food choices. It's not melodramatic to say, as others have pointed out, that our food choices are life and death decisions. Would you intentionally eat a small, non-lethal amount of arsenic or cyanide each day, even though it may taste good? Probably not, but you could well be one of millions who willingly take in toxic foods that will over time have the same effect, and it all starts with just one bite, with one decision you make in the moment.

Eat now, pay later. Or change your eating now, and your investment will be rewarded many times over.

Just as your thoughts happen now, your feelings happen now, your experiences of all kinds happen now, and not in the past or the future, so do your food choices. You do not know what choices you will make later today, or tomorrow, but you can have control over what you put into your mouth right now. Or don't. This is not a "just for today" program, since you don't know what you will do later today. None of us does. But you have control, if you wish to take it, over what you do right now.

And please don't fall into the trap of deciding never to eat such and such a thing ever again. Did you ever make a New Year's resolution? Did you stick with it? One part of you, one side of you, may make a resolution, and you can always count on another part of you that wants nothing to do with the resolution, breaking it. That part writes the check, and the rest of you pays the price.

Food choices are the same way. You make them in the moment, and by thinking you are giving things up for good, you are only deluding yourself and setting yourself up for failure. Because the desire and the craving for that particular food you are "giving up forever" will reassert itself, in spades, when you least expect it.

So, right here and right now, make the following declaration to yourself, and put this at the top of your list of the benefits you will gain by changing your eating: "I make my food choices in the here and now."

Let's talk about some more about uncontrolled eating, from a slightly different point of view. Again, you don't hear about people pigging out on broccoli or quinoa, do you? No, with few exceptions, we pig out on other types of foods.

- Processed foods.

- Restaurant foods.

- Colas and soft drinks.

- Certain home cooked foods.

As we spoke of, the hunger that is natural can be satisfied, but addictive hunger is insatiable. Feeding food cravings by eating is like giving liquor to an alcoholic or more drugs to a junkie—they always want more.

Certainly we have this instinctive need to eat, which must be dealt with, but it doesn't have to be the burden that it now is since we so often never allow ourselves to experience it.

Food craving, as you now know, is a combination of an intense physical desire, as well as a psychological obsession. You think constantly about food. You salivate at the thought. The incessantly repeating thought. Not the same thing as hunger, by a long shot.

So what is the solution? How do we lay aside all that went before and really find a new direction? We have to change our thinking, plus we need to direct what we consider to be food to another realm. And not go back.

Easy to say, more difficult to do.

Like we discussed, we need to include in what we eat things that are naturally low in the unhealthy stuff, but which deliver a lot of flavor, as well as vitamins, minerals, fiber, and so on. We are talking, as I have said before, about a plant-based diet. Whole foods, plant based, no added oil. Foods using these are low in calories, low in fat, high in vitamins and micronutrients, minerals, and fiber, instead of the reverse, which are the high fat high calorie nutrient poor things.

13. Deprivation
(Or, "I can't eat this...")

As we touched briefly earlier, one of the things we run up against in embracing a new way of eating is the feeling of deprivation. So let's go into it a bit deeper.

Deprivation makes us feel that we will be lacking something, that something will be missing, or more particularly, that something is being taken away. Something in us often feels that because when embarking down the path of whole food plant based eating, we are somehow deprived of the things we are giving up.

Or if we start thinking these thoughts of "not being able to have certain foods" (for this is how we frame it), it's like when someone tells you to not think about pink elephants. What do you think of? Pink elephants, of course.

And if we tell ourselves we "can't have" certain foods, we see and think of a cornucopia of hamburgers, pizzas, potato chips, and our other favorites, drifting through our minds and emotions, and endlessly repeating.

So let's examine this.

The words and phrases we tell ourselves are very important in this, because we believe what we constantly and consistently repeat. Whether true or not. Let's revisit this more detail.

We usually say something to ourselves like, "I can't have this particular food". What happens when you tell a two year old that he can't have something? Of course, he wants it even more and it can become an obsession. Sadly, we haven't really progressed from this mentality of a two year old, unless we shed light on what is going on.

If we stop eating steak and fries for health reasons, by choosing to throw our weight in a healthy direction, are we really being deprived of these foods? Or is it just the voices inside us, our Evil Twin, with the familiar siren cry, because we have old feelings coming to the surface in the form of words it can work with, words of deprivation, words of "I can't have these foods?" In reality, we're not being deprived of anything at all. We are adding to our lives, we are adding to our health, we are adding to our wellbeing.

Certainly, everyone has choice in this, if they want to take it on. They can choose to eat whatever they want. They really are not being deprived. Eat now, pay later.

But if you are smart, you may choose to avoid the steaks and ice cream for the greater good of your health, weight, and wellbeing. This is called "throwing your weight", because there is always a yes and a no to throw your weight behind.

Right now, I am sorry to say, as you are, you have literally no choice in the matter; there is no "yes" or "no," there is only the automatic face-feeding that's gotten you into so much trouble up to this point. And it is much harder to feel deprived when you truly feel you have choice in the matter of what to eat. You do have a choice, whether you want to accept it or not. Although, admittedly, you may not always feel that way! You do have choice. And there will always be a struggle between the "yes" and the "no."

What you will do, in a moment of choice? Nobody knows. Maybe you will decide to stay on, or to get onto, the path of healthy eating; maybe not. Healthy eating is always a moment by moment decision.

After a while, after new eating habits are established, it will become a whole lot easier, and at some point can become second nature, but right now, unless you are really able to draw a line in the sand, there may be an inner struggle each time you eat.

14. The "Cheat Day"
(Just don't tell your husband or wife!)

Some diets or eating plans include a "cheat day." This eating plan is not one of them. If you are thinking like this, like you need a cheat day, you are feeling deprived, or are lying to yourself, or think you can somehow beat the addiction with this little trick.

Eating healthy is additive, it isn't a deprivation, and again, if you look at it this way, it can help. In fact, the more you can remind yourself how helpful and beneficial healthy eating can be, the easier it will be to deal with desires to eat, and cravings as well. And the notion of a cheat day will make less and less sense to you.

Thinking you "deserve" a cheat day, to reward yourself for some imagined virtue, is a clue that at least a part of your thinking is haywire, and this part will get you into deep trouble.

But let's talk about this idea of a cheat day. Your body doesn't take a day off on a cheat day. Your heart doesn't take a day off, nor does your digestive system, nor any other body part, nor does the sun, or any other part of the world of nature. Nor does a food addiction. The notion of a cheat day is an imaginary construct, as if it would make something new into something easier. Any feeling of a need for a day off from an eating plan is strictly in your head. Not only do you not need it, it will undermine and eventually destroy all your other efforts.

Let's talk about a cheat day from the point of view of overeating addictively all these salt, sugar, and fat-laden foods. What is the key to successfully overcoming addictive behavior? We talked about it: total abstinence from the addictive substance, and allowing time to heal you from the cravings.

If you want to quit smoking, do you give yourself a cheat day? If you are an alcoholic, and you want to quit drinking, do you give yourself a cheat day? What happens if you do? As surely as night follows day, you eventually go back to smoking or drinking.

We can look at it from another point of view: if you are married or in a relationship, is it OK if your spouse has a cheat day, that one day a week he or she is free to do whatever comes naturally (or unnaturally, as the case may be) with anyone he or she wants, other than you? I didn't think so.

There is a little thing called "commitment" which is lacking in all these examples. And in the notion of a cheat day. It's a sort of back door reservation you are giving yourself that under certain circumstances you will allow yourself to backslide. You have your fingers crossed behind your back if you are thinking like this.

You will be FAR better off drawing a line in the sand, one that you do not cross, come what may, instead of giving yourself any sort of an "out." Even if you from time to time fall short!

Let's say you have a difficult day at work, or you get into a fight with your spouse. What's to keep you from deciding to have your cheat day that day? Nothing, this is just another one of the many, many numbers our ET runs on us. He, or she, signs the checks, and we pay. Plus, do you honestly think you won't take your regularly scheduled cheat day as well?

Let's talk about this cheat day from another perspective. What if once a week you somehow actually get away with this, keeping your weight and eating at a maintenance level without the rest of your eating plan collapsing. Do you think you might go overboard and eat an extra 500 or 1000 calories on that day? Odds are it would be more, since you'd be making up for lost time, right? But if you took in ONLY 500 or 1000 extra calories per cheat day, assuming a cheat day once a week, that works out to a mere 26,000 or 52,000 extra calories per year, or 7.5 to 15 pounds you'd gain in a year. In ten years that's 75 pounds or 150 pounds you've gained, or will not have lost, by having a cheat day. Who is really getting cheated here?

So there will be times you REALLY want to fall off the wagon. To "cheat," so to speak. You feel the temptations are just so overwhelming that "just this once" you will "cheat." Which isn't really possible as we have seen, but something in you will try to convince you that it is possible. So let's look at this temptation, another way, from the point of view of an idea, since we may backslide at some point. For nothing in life goes in a straight line.

We decide to drive to California: we have to zig and zag, go through some pretty unpleasant places, and if we stick with it, eventually we will wind up in California. The roads are never totally straight. At times with our eating plan we may follow an equally indirect route. At times, we just want to hang it up. To say forget about it. To come back to where we started. We may backslide.

This can happen in the transition to healthy eating. This change doesn't necessarily go in a straight line. And our thought process and emotional situation isn't always the same—it's not always positive and enthusiastic. We experience constant inner change. Sometimes we can get pretty negative about healthy eating!

You also may have some physical zigging and zagging in the form of withdrawal symptoms. These can be headaches, fatigue, crankiness, or a general feeling of falling off the wagon. And you will have this emotional zigging and zagging as well. Does this mean you are permanently and forever screwed, doomed to a lifetime of overeating? Of course not, but you must immediately get back on the horse, or the wagon, depending on the metaphor you are using. Like right now. In the moment. Immediately. Forget the beguiling voice of your ET that says, "Today's shot to hell. I messed up. I'll get back on the wagon tomorrow." If it's not possible to do it immediately, get back on the eating plan as soon as possible.

If you give in, and then give up, you are giving up on yourself, and that's the worst thing you can possibly give up on. And the longer you binge, the harder it is to end. Addictive behavior of any kind often doesn't move in a straight line. Many people backslide, so please be a little forgiving of yourself for being human!

The voice of the ET may now enter and say something like, "Well, since it's a normal part of the process, I might as well have some ice cream." This is a voice that comes from the addiction, from five percent truth and the rest lies, as are all the negative thoughts and feelings that come from addiction. They are just the voices of temptation.

As are the voices that beg and plead for a "cheat" day!

15. Silence is Golden
(So shaddup, already!)

Is there anything more ubiquitous in the world than opinions? Everyone's got 'em! Opinions on the weather, on politics, on religion, on what we should do or not do, how we should behave, and so on.

And some are really strong trigger points. We get really emotional about things like religion, politics, and health. Particularly on diet, everybody has opinions, whether right or wrong. Everybody is the expert. Just ask them. YOU have opinions on diet! We ALL do!

These opinions on diet aren't limited to you, or other members of the general public; they abound among medical professionals, governmental officials, and diet book authors. What's the healthiest diet? What diet will help you lose weight best? What diet will help you keep it off?

Sadly, much of it is another example of the blind leading the blind. With all the accumulated "wisdom" of the experts, and more medical knowledge than at any time in known history, we still have, as you know, two thirds of the people in this country being overweight or obese.

Why is this? Well, the reasons are many and complex, but let's abridge and simplify it a bit in the following way: one, there are a lot of people out there that really don't know what they are talking about, as we discussed. "It's what they know that just ain't so," to paraphrase Mark Twain, like we discussed earlier.

And two, even if someone has the correct, accurate, and even actionable information, it is very difficult to take, and to maintain, consistent action because of the world we live in and the power of habit.

Regarding the first group, the people who don't know what they are talking about, even though they think they do, they are always going to be there. There is still the Flat Earth Society. There are people who think we really never landed on the moon. There are people who still revere Adolf Hitler, and there are still people who think that if you aren't a white person, you are a non-human subspecies, and hopefully their numbers continue to dwindle!

Certainly there are people in the first group that have ideas about diet which, although they may help you lose weight, either do it in a way that isn't healthy, or that set you up for regaining the weight at the end. It's what they know that isn't so. Again, the idea here is not about going on a diet, it's about changing what you eat, about changing your lifestyle, so not only are you able to lose weight in a healthy manner, but you are able to keep it off as well.

So what's a person to do, if you decide to adopt the whole foods plant based eating style? If you start sharing about what you are doing with other people, you are going to become an opinion magnet! And a negative opinion magnet, at that. You will bring out the inner "expert" from the person you are speaking to.

Everyone will have something to say as to how you should lead your life. And how to eat. And things will get more confusing than they are already. My guess is that you can verify this from your own experience, if you've ever dieted—the first thing people want to do is to talk about THEIR diet, right?

If you mention you are avoiding meat, you'll attract questions about where do you get your protein, which we've covered. Same thing with milk, since most people think, wrongly, that every body needs milk. Where do you get your calcium? (from greens, actually, and from many other things as well). Same with fish: where do you get your Omega 3s? (flax and nuts—plenty!) But if you are a hardcore meat eater, you are never asked where you get your fiber.

The only sensible question you will be asked is about where you get your vitamin B12. And a simple daily supplement gives you what you need, so make sure you take this, when you start eating this way.

You will be regaled with stories about someone who ate nothing but plants, and to whom horrible things happened. You'll get cautionary suggestions, there will be temptations to eat other things that never would have been offered had you not mentioned you were avoiding certain foods, and so on. Is this helpful? Can getting bombarded with what is essentially negativity help you change the way you eat? Or are these really thinly disguised efforts to drag YOU back within the comfort zone of the other person?

Because if you talk about your change of eating, you represent a challenge to the status quo, you will force another person to question the intelligence of what he or she is eating, and even though they won't come out and say so, that makes people extremely uncomfortable.

The best thing to do in social situations is just to keep a preemptive silence as much as possible. Don't bring attention to yourself. If someone comments about your not taking a bagel and cream cheese (at somewhere around 370 calories, by the way) at an office meeting, you can say you had a big breakfast, or you don't really want one, or you have packed a big lunch and don't want to spoil your appetite, or that you are avoiding this sort of thing for a day or two to see how it affects you. And this is true, we don't know what choices we will make in the future.

There is no need to explain yourself to other people, even though we often feel we must. So say what you need to say in terms the other person can understand and relate to. As succinctly as possible. Then change the subject.

Whatever you do, please don't say you've totally changed what you eat and are dining on exclusively whole food plant based things from now on! For you don't know, any more than I do, what the next meal—or the next temptation—may bring. And you will be putting a huge bull's-eye for the other person's resentment and ill will right between your eyes or on the seat of your pants!

Telling someone you're changing how you eat is also very difficult to do without a tone of voice creeping in that smacks of superiority and of one-upmanship. I'm sure you've had other people do this to you. Please don't do it to others, as the reaction will be far less than favorable!

The other thing is, silence keeps your eating affirmations to yourself. It's your decision what you eat, or don't eat. If you start eating in the healthy way just to be seen by others, you are making your lifestyle change for the real or imagined opinions of others, instead of for yourself.

Let's say you change your eating for the sake of your husband or wife. The moment you get mad at your partner, you'll have a perfect excuse to start pigging out, out of spite. (You'll "fix them", right?) But, if you change your eating strictly for yourself, no matter how mad you may get at your partner, it will be harder to be vindictive if your choices are for you, and not for him or her.

If you go to a party, usually there are things you will want to eat that will be healthy, or at least reasonably so. There is very often a veggie platter with hummus, baba ganoush, or some such thing. My favorite strategy is to eat before I go there, so the temptations aren't overwhelming. You are there to see your friends, aren't you? Or are you there just to eat?

If you go to a potluck, it's a whole lot easier. Bring something that you will like and that's healthy. Most people will not be paying attention to what you eat. And bring plenty in case you wind up eating your own food exclusively!

If you inadvertently let something slip about your new way of eating, and the conversation starts going down a path you don't want it to, simply change direction by asking the person you are with a question about themself. I've used this trick on many occasions and under many circumstances, since people always want to talk about their favorite subject: themselves. And in a flash, they will forget your new way of eating.

There is another aspect to silence that we can include here as well: keeping inner silence as much as possible. This is even more difficult, if not impossible, believe it or not, than keeping silent in front of others. If and when you catch yourself thinking about junk foods, about how wonderful and delicious they are, and so on, remind yourself of what they really do to you in terms of health and weight, and make the effort to change your inner channel to other thoughts. We all tend to be indulgent in our thought process, and here is a great opportunity to go against that, when possible.

Similarly, stay away as much as possible from exposing yourself to TV and other media ads about foods. They don't have your best interest at heart, and they can start your thought process going in a way that won't help you. That's what they're designed to do, after all.

So keep it to yourself. You don't need to share what you are doing with other people, you don't need to expose yourself to advertising influences. They said to me in AA: "keep the plug in the jug." I'm suggesting as far as food is concerned that you keep the plug in your mug. You do not need to talk about what you are doing. There is no requirement, social or otherwise, to do so. You do not have to justify your choices, no matter how you may feel otherwise in the moment. If you are with friends, you can be at the event simply to enjoy their company. You don't need to say, "Look at me." You can lead by silent example, and after you are a little farther along, and have lost weight, and people ask you, you can start to share a bit at a time. And don't forget to recommend this book!

Conclusion

As we've seen, we need to go a new direction with our eating. A solution to this morass (pun intended) we find ourselves in. A direction toward a whole, fresh non-processed low fat diet without animal proteins, which is what we as human beings ate for most of our existence. A way of eating that does not ignite and excite these cravings for foods that our bodies have been trained to go after by both the food industry and our own indulgences.

We are in the middle, not of an obesity epidemic, but a food addiction epidemic, and the obesity and weight gain is the result of the problem. It is not the problem itself, although most people think it is. And the solution is to change what we eat to a more traditional diet, consisting mostly if not entirely of plant based whole foods, with a minimum, if not the total exclusion, of added oil.

The native diets where people live the longest use this formula. This isn't some newly invented, odd fad diet that I've come up with; it's been around since the beginning of humanity. It's the normal, natural diet that most people ate most of the time, with the exception of kings, royalty, and the wealthy, and kings, royalty, and the wealthy were the people who developed the health problems we now have.

And there are a few areas in the world where people still eat in the traditional way.

The old Okinawans, for example followed the way of eating that I am advocating. Minimal animal protein, lots of sweet potatoes, rice and veggies. There are many others.

There are a number of areas in the world with life expectancies going over 90, and in fact, there is one now in Southern California (see The Blue Zones, referenced in the Resources section). It's not confined to backwoods parts of the world. We can have our own version of the same thing wherever we happen to be: delicious, healthy, and allowing the body to return to a sensible, realistic weight for itself, and probably increasing our life expectancies as well.

As we have seen, this isn't a regimen of carrot and celery sticks with a side of brown rice. The entire plant kingdom is at your disposal, and the food can be absolutely incredible!

As we've discussed, let none think that this eating plan has been created to enable them to get into a size seven dress, or to look good for a wedding. That may happen, it may not, but it's not my focus. If you want to become a sex object, that's not what this is about. It's about helping you to get to a sane, healthy weight that is right for your particular body and body type, not about recreating you into someone else's fantasy about what the ideal body type is. And that's doomed to fail at the outset because the goal is unrealistic. This may come as a shock, but you are never again going to have the body of a seventeen year old.

Unless, of course, you happen to be seventeen!

And this plan of eating will, after a few weeks, virtually eliminate food cravings, as long as you don't nibble, or tempt fate with the lie of "just one bite," or a cheat day. They really do dwindle over time.

But for right now, remember that added sugar, salt and fat, particularly in processed foods, are what set the cravings into motion, creating a nearly irresistible compulsion that you will not be able to satisfy by eating. Eating then becomes a futile attempt to avoid the temporary discomfort of not eating. You cannot put out a fire by pouring gasoline on it, and you can't stop food cravings by continuing to try to control your eating of junk and processed foods. How can you possibly expect them to go away by giving yourself the very things that are causing them in the first place?

A Word From the Author

There you have it! You have a basic, though pretty comprehensive introduction to why dieting doesn't work, the forces working against change in our world, how you can end your food cravings, an intro into the idea of food addiction and cravings, and lots of tips and strategies for adopting a new lifestyle based on whole foods, plant based eating.

My wish for you is that reading this book is the first step toward your regaining control of your eating, your weight, and your life. And in fact, any of the eating plans suggested in the books in the resources will work for you. I will be creating my own methods for taking this further, in addition to other books in the works, but for right now I need to refer you to others.

Also, now that this book is completed, I've started work on a subsequent book. You'll be learning about—among other things—more about the myth that we need to get our protein from animal products, the feelings of not having enough time to eat healthily, changing our eating habits, overcoming our own personal inner objections to this new way of eating, dealing with friends and family who may not be responsive to this new way of eating, and actually making the transition to this way of eating—gradually or all at once.

And you may rediscover—or discover, as the case may be, the joys of cooking for yourself. And how to have time to do this!

Many people know that whole foods plant based eating is healthiest, but the obstacles to getting from here to there seem too formidable to attempt to conquer. This new book, and subsequent works, will address how to overcome these.

The first step in any new direction is education, and by having read this, you have begun yours. You can continue your education by downloading five FREE smoothie recipes (including the infamous Carrot Cake Smoothie recipe)—just go to www.CurbThoseCravings.com/five-free-recipes.

This website will put you in touch with other materials as well: I will be addressing many issues that haven't been addressed in this book: accountability, help, new ideas, recipes and so on. This website and information feed is a work in progress, so please join us, to stay up to date on new books—and also so you can get helpful and informative items on your diet and health.

Also make sure you take advantage of the items in the "Resources" section, as there is tons of information—much of it free--there as well.

Thank you so much for reading to the end! And if you enjoyed this book, please tell your friends, so they may gain the benefit of reading it too. Remember, go to www.CurbThoseCravings.com/five-free-recipes to get your free recipes, and to keep the material coming to you. And much of it will be free!

Al Davis
P.O. Box 79032
Belmont MA 02479

www.CurbThoseCravings.com

Resources

(Yes, there is lots of scientific evidence to back up what I'm saying, and plenty of places to get more info and help)

Book List

There are tons of books on the subject of weight loss, some better, some worse, and most are pretty terrible. But these are some of the ones I've found most helpful, because they focus on lifestyle, not weight. All are generally available on Amazon, often available for as little as a penny plus $3.99 shipping. Such a deal!

If money is a problem, many if not all of these books and videos should be available free or at very low cost from your library.

The China Study, by Colin Campbell, PhD. A huge study undertaken in China, comparing the diets and the results of different diets on the Chinese population. The results are startling: the people who ate like we do in this country, with an emphasis on meat, fish, and dairy have the same problems with being overweight and the other health complications of our western style diet, but those who ate a more traditional Chinese diet of mostly vegetables, rice and fruit had virtually no such problems. Also, you will be amazed as to what Dr. Campbell discovered about milk!

The End of Overeating, by David Kessler, MD. Kessler is the former head of the FDA, who blew the whistle on the tobacco industry, and here is beginning to do the same with the food industry. This is a good—and easy to read—intro to the effects of sugar, salt and fat, and how they affect our eating.

Sugar, Salt and Fat: How The Food Giants Hooked Us, by Michael Moss. An investigative report from a Pulitzer Prize winning journalist into the topic. More detailed than the Kessler book, frightening, and interesting. If you thought I was exaggerating about food addictions and what food companies are doing to create them, this may change your thinking. And help change your eating as well.

The Spectrum, by Dr. Dean Ornish (in fact, any book by Dean Ornish). His approach is very similar to mine, it is highly successful for weight loss, and it's recommended. Includes recipes.

The Pleasure Trap, by Doug Lisle. If you think you are weak and undisciplined because of being overweight, this can help. You don't need to beat yourself up any more. Lots of good material, and there is plenty to learn from him.

Eat to Live, and *The Starch Solution*, both by Joel Fuhrman, M.D.—and in fact, any book by him. Also similar, also highly recommended. Lots of recipes.

The Engine 2 Diet, by Rip Esselstyn. How a change in their meat-eating ways helped a bunch of Austin firefighters not only lose lots of weight, but get healthier. Recipes included, very easy ones at that. This is the same Engine 2 that's being promoted by Whole Foods right now as a product line.

My Beef With Meat, by the same author, has a very good discussion on why eating meat is not only bad for your health, but has other horrible consequences as well. And you will learn far more about protein than most people on the planet now know.

The Healthiest Diet on the Planet, by Dr. John & Mary McDougall—and any other book by them as well. Shows you how you can not only lose weight, but prevent disease, look younger, and feel your best through eating foods you love—pizza, pancakes, potatoes, pasta, and much more. Includes recipes.

The Power Of Habit, by Charles Duhigg, explaining how and why habits exist, and how to change them. Has a good focus on weight loss, and creating new habits around healthy eating. A must-read if you wish to change your habits around food.

Mindless Eating, by Brian Wansink, exploring why we eat far more than we think—and monkey wrenches we can throw into our works to reverse this situation. Intelligent and entertaining, highly recommended.

Slim By Design, also by Brian Wansink, exploring more about the mindless eating we all do, and specific rituals we can add into our habit-filled lives to make healthy choices habitual, instead of something we have to struggle mightily to achieve.

How Not To Die, by Michael Greger MD. Nowhere nearly as glum as the title, this book gives the main causes of death in the US, most of which are brought on (and curable) by lifestyle. Highly recommended, and you ignore this book at your peril.

A Plant Based Life, the transition to a whole foods plant based life, the benefits and obstacles, by Micaela Cook Karlsen. Well written, highly informative and useful. Includes lots of really good recipes, including one by me!

*Meat is for P*****S*, by John Joseph, available on Kindle. Look up by author's name on Amazon, you'll find the book. Leader of punk rock group Cro Magnon, John geared this book toward men and the attitudes we as men often have toward not eating meat. Written in an "in your face" style, sort of as one of your locker room buddies might tell you. Nothing effete about this book, that's for sure!

Cookbooks and Cooking Resources

In addition to the recipes in some of the books above, here are some cookbooks and resources I've found helpful. You say you're not a cook? Remember, you don't need to be a five star chef to be a healthy cook. Just find ten or fifteen easy and recipes you like—or more, or fewer—and that's all you really need to start. Unless, of course, you are like me, and try new things all the time!

Remember that, like in all cookbooks, there will be good—and not so good—recipes. I have been cooking for over sixty years, and at this point I'm pretty competent at it, so I do know what I'm talking about when recommending cookbooks. Most of the recipes I've pulled out of these I would consider anywhere from good to excellent—but peoples' tastes are different. You may not like things I like, and vise versa. (I can't stand tofu, for example!)

And when you are starting a new way of eating, it may take getting used to—or not. Believe me, you can get used to anything, if you are motivated—and fortunately, a whole foods plant based way of eating can be absolutely delicious and for many will need no transition time at all!

The Happy Herbivore, by Lindsay Nixon. And any other books by the same author. Extremely easy and tasty veggie recipes with no added fat. See also www.happyherbivore.com for more recipes, and she also sells meal plans for those of you who are on the go. I've gotten lots of keeper recipes from her.

She also has written a terrific—and highly recommended—book on the transition to whole foods plant based eating (with recipes) called *The Happy Herbivore Guide To Plant Based Eating*.

Also, check out her podcast: "Shortcut To Slim", where she tackles the problems of whole foods plant based weight loss from a science based perspective. Intelligent and thorough.

Bravo, by Ramses Bravo. These recipes come from the True North Health Center in Santa Rosa, California, started by Dr. Doug Lisle referenced above. The recipes are generally very good, although more complicated than the ones by Lindsay, so don't take on a recipe from here unless you have a bit more time and skill than just beginner.

Forks Over Knives Cookbook, by Del Stroufe. Generally good recipes, although rather complicated, and I've gotten some keepers out of here too.

Forks Over Knives iPhone App: good stuff here as well, easy recipes, includes the ability to add a shopping list, plus a place to add notes. Also available for Android. This is the one

I use most. They are constantly updating it with new recipes, too.

Helpful app: *Happy Cow* will help you find plant-based vegan, vegetarian, restaurants with vegan options, and supermarkets in a particular area.

The *Yelp* app will do the same, just enter "vegan" and "present location" to find what's near you. You might be surprised—and hopefully pleasantly!

21 Day Vegan Kickstart, an app from the Physicians Committee for responsible medicine. This is a free app to get you started in the whole foods plant based direction.

www.Meetup.com should have plenty of vegan and plant-friendly Meetups available. Look also for raw foods groups. They have an app, or you can find them on line. Don't, though, assume that because someone is vegan that they are also a healthy eater!

And there are plenty of other apps as well for whole foods plant based eating. Just search the app store under "vegan".

Movies

These are all available on Netflix or from Amazon, and many are available at your library.

Forks Over Knives. The premise is that we can avoid the knife of the surgeon through what we put onto our forks. If you watch no other movie, watch this one—it's a real eye opener. You'll see people who have lost a bunch of weight, and gotten rid of other chronic health problems to boot. Watch this first! And you can find this free on line and on Netflix, as of this writing.

Plant Pure Nation, by the producers of Forks Over Knives, starring Nelson Campbell MD, the son of one of the co-authors of the China Study, exposing the incredible influence of the food lobby on the lawmaking process, and the very real effects on a small town in middle America, where a bunch of people switch to a low fat whole food plant based diet. With very real and extremely beneficial consequences. Available on Amazon, and as of this writing on Netflix.

Fat, Sick And Nearly Dead. Although I'm not an advocate of juicing as a weight reduction strategy, the transformation of the two men in this film is remarkable. Well worth seeing!

The Engine 2 Kitchen Rescue. Entertaining purge of toxic—and not atypical—kitchens by Rip Esselstyn, showing you how to do it. You will be amazed how much toxic stuff is in an average home—and not just underneath the kitchen sink!

Vegucated. How three meat and potatoes New Yorkers switched to a healthier diet, and the results of it. Entertaining and informative. It doesn't follow the plan I'm recommending, but watching the struggle of the people involved is fascinating and revealing.

Hungry for Change. Excellent movie on food addiction and what the food industry does to us, totally beneath our radar.

Cowspiracy. Did you know that the amount of water required to produce a hamburger would be enough for you to take a shower for two months? This movie is a fascinating look at how the meat and dairy industries are keeping the information secret on what the environmental impact of factory farming is, both here, and around the world. Highly recommended—unless you like having your head in the sand.

Supersize Me! Amazing movie about a guy who ate at McDonalds three times per day, and the consequences he suffered, ranging from massive weight gain to psychological difficulties—and impotence. Yikes!

Also, nutritionist Jeff Novik has a whole bunch of instructional videos on a variety of topics, ranging from general education on plant based eating to many, many VERY easy and quick to prepare dishes using a lot of frozen and canned ingredients (yes, there are really healthy versions of these, and he names the names. Some of Jeff's material is free. See http://www.jeffnovick.com/RD/Home.html).

Useful website: www.nutritionfacts.org Weekly (or more) free videos and essays on various health topics, all centered around food, many on obesity. Sign up, search the database, get regular short videos on health and nutrition—free!

Meal Plans

In addition to the very excellent ones being sold by www.HappyHerbivore.com (she'll give a free sample, by the way), also see:

www.PlantPlate.com, they have a 28 day plan, the food for which will cost around five bucks a day. So much for this being an expensive way to eat! See http://tinyurl.com/joeyvvj to order.

Free meal plan, through Dr. Michael Greger, author of <u>How Not To Die</u>, and founder of Nutritionfacts.org. See http://tinyurl.com/gtqcg62/. Read the article, go to the meal plan. They have the free one, and two paid ones.

About the Author

Al's life can hardly been seen as having gone in a straight line.

Quite the antithesis!

After reclaiming his life and health following stopping smoking, drinking, drugs and addictive overeating—not to mention conquering chronic depression—over 35 years ago, Al—while doing lots of other stuff—has delved ever more deeply into the questions of healthy eating and diet, and how we can apply them to our own lives.

Following the recent illnesses and deaths of several friends, he decided it was time to bring into the world what he had discovered about not only weight loss, but about the tremendous effect that what we eat has on not just our health, but our emotional well-being as well.

Over the last 35 years, he has become an inspirational speaker, has written another book besides this one, has written essays, poems, and theater pieces, is now an accomplished home chef, has earned his second degree black belt in karate, speaks two foreign languages, has traveled all over the USA and Europe, plus visited Egypt, Peru, Mexico and Central America—and while there, sought out the healthiest and tastiest foods in each of those places. He has lived in Italy, Munich, and London, in addition to many places in the USA.

He is also a real estate investor, and has been self-employed for the last 35 years.

He is a graduate of Earlham College, in Richmond, Indiana, and has done further study at New York University and the London School of Economics.

If he can do all this stuff as an ex-drunk, what's holding YOU back? Find out what he has learned can help *you*. Start now, by getting your five FREE whole foods plant based recipes—including his infamous Carrot Cake Smoothie recipe, and take the first step toward transforming your life! Just go to www.CurbThoseCravings.com.

He resides currently in Belmont, Massachusetts.

A Special and Urgent Request!!!

Thank you for reading this book, and I hope you found value in it as well.

I really appreciate your feedback, since it helps me improve the book.

So please, let me know what you think, so I can make it better and better, both for you, as well as for subsequent readers.

Therefore...

Kindly leave me a helpful and honest review on Amazon. Thank you so much!

—Al Davis

How This Book Came to Be
(From gathering dust, to a real, live book)

This book only existed as a series of unpublished essays, which languished alone, untouched, on a shelf, for over a year. Then I discovered Self-Publishing School, and the whole thing turned around. If you think you have the makings of a book, either inside yourself or in partially written form, please check out the videos in the link on the next page. May your healthy eating and your writing adventures proceed at the same time!

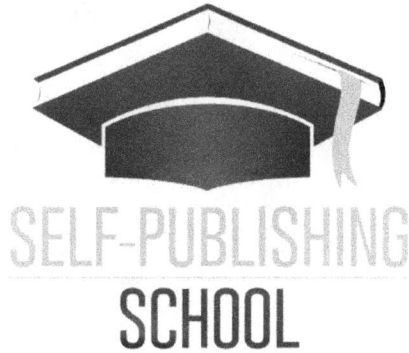